DR.
SOLOMON'S
EASY, NO-RISK
DIET

DR. SOLOMON'S EASY, NO-RISK DIET

by
Neil Solomon, M.D. Ph.D.
and
Mary Knudson

COWARD, McCANN & GEOGHEGAN, INC.
New York

Second Impression

Copyright © 1974 by Neil Solomon, M.D., Ph.D.
All rights reserved. This book, or parts thereof, may not be reproduced in any form without permission in writing from the publisher. Published on the same day in Canada by Longman Canada Limited, Toronto.
SBN: 698-10599-0
Library of Congress Catalog Card Number: 73-93766
Printed in the United States of America

Chapter Ten appeared in abridged form in *Retirement Living*, Copyright © 1974 by Neil Solomon and Mary Knudson.

AUTHOR'S NOTE

Pertinent scientific data used in this book have been published in medical journals (see For Further Reading) or have been accepted for publication in the *Maryland State Medical Journal.*

I have made a few changes in my patients' case study circumstances in order to prevent any possible identification of or embarrassment to them.

DEDICATION

N.S. dedicates this book to his most lovable and understanding family. N.S. also dedicates this book to his mother, Clara, and father Max, who gave him good genes and good values.

And M.K. dedicates this book to her mother, Anne, a beautiful person.

Both authors dedicate this book to all those people who want good, solid nutrition, and to everyone trying to get on top of their problems.

ACKNOWLEDGMENTS

The author is indebted to Mrs. Janette Martin, Director of the Nutrition Department of the Johns Hopkins Hospital, for her invaluable nutrition consultation. Mrs. Martin is a highly respected nutritionist, and she took much care to help me give the diet as much variety as possible, yet keep it well balanced nutritionally. The author, with gratitude, thanks Patricia Brehaut Soliman for her superb editing. The author also thanks his wife, Frema Solomon, for her dietary editing, inspiration and patience.

The author would also like to acknowledge with gratitude the following professionals who reviewed the manuscript: Theodore E. Woodward, MD, Professor and Head of the Department of Medicine, University of Maryland Hospital, Baltimore. Thurman Mott, Jr., MD, Assistant Professor of the School of Medicine, University of Maryland, Baltimore. James H. Bready, book columnist, *The Sunday Sun*, Baltimore. Gerald Walker, the New York *Times*, and Margaret C. Pergrem, Welch Medical Library, Johns Hopkins University, Baltimore.

And, of course, special gratitude to my many patients for their help and encouragement.

CONTENTS

DR.

SOLOMON'S

EASY, NO-RISK

DIET

INTRODUCTION

Two years ago I wrote *The Truth About Weight Control,* a book that assembled in one place all the background, *theoretical* information you need for permanent weight control. Over the following twenty-four months, as I worked with patients, lectured, debated diet faddists on television talk shows, and saw the maze of articles and books on crash diets flood the supermarkets and magazine racks, one thing became dramatically apparent to me—something that badly needed remedying—the faulty information the public was being fed about fad diets. I was serious about trying to neutralize the misinformation being disseminated by the "fat doctor" talk show experts. It was in this concerned frame of mind that I agreed to debate publicly—and have repeatedly debated—leading proponents of fad diets.

But telling people what *not* to do only meets their diet

dilemma halfway. Many people I met through my discussions of nutrition urged me to provide them with a safe but effective diet, and it was in response to their need that I decided to write this book. The diet described here is more than just a diet—it's a way of life that is easy to follow, safe, nutritionally sound, and will result first in weight loss and then lead into a trim figure-keeping program for you for the rest of your life.

If you are a fat person who doesn't like being fat but finds it hard to lose weight permanently, this may be the most important book you will ever read. While I don't profess to have a miracle, one-of-its-kind diet, I do think the diet I offer is the most interesting and varied well-balanced diet you'll ever try. And you *will* lose weight on it. It has proved successful, easy and as risk-free as any general reducing diet can be. The point is—good nutrition means eating a well-balanced diet from the four food groups, regardless of whether you are on a diet to lose weight, gain weight, or maintain your weight.

I also teach you how to tone up your mind to discipline yourself to stay on the diet—the gentle art of Diet Meditation.

It should help you to remember this single thing: You are not alone in needing to diet. Four out of ten Americans are overweight. Dieting is simply knowing what you eat and selecting wisely. And it is not only fat people who need to watch their diet. While you may avoid a serving of potato salad because of the mayonnaise and potatoes, your slender neighbor may also shun it simply because he has trouble digesting green peppers. While chocolate may cry calories at you, it may give as many anxious moments to the teen-ager or young adult worried about complexion problems.

A lot of fat people are probably the victims of mothers who overfed them as children, offering food in lieu of love—mothers who found it quicker and easier to pop a bottle into a crying infant's mouth than to take time to hold and talk and cuddle. Later the problem was fostered, as mother misguidedly handed out sweet treats to comfort her children's hurt moments or to reward them.

How many times in your adult life have you gone on an eating binge when you were emotionally upset? Was this a subconscious return to the way you were comforted when you were a baby? We'll talk more about this and about how to handle the psychological you, as well as the physical you, later in the book. One thing we know for sure: milk is no substitute for love. Neither is any other food.

This book is dedicated to helping us love ourselves and each other. And you will love yourself more when you are thin than when you are fat. Remember, you need never apologize or feel embarrassed for passing up something others are eating. You are the master of your body and you help determine its shape—and *you can be the architect of its lasting good health.*

I have great concern about the risks and recklessness of fad diets and would like first to discuss that with you.

1

THE PERILS

OF FAD DIETS

Shortcuts can be tempting. If you're fat, you may feel that a diet should have one purpose—to make you lose weight as fast as possible. In this frame of mind you'll probably keep searching for the latest "big promise-little work" diet plan you can find.

Q. What's wrong with the popular crash fad diets?
A. What's wrong with shaking hands with an octopus? Or swimming a long distance on a full stomach, or roasting your marshmallow on a toothpick or taking an overdose of sleeping pills? *You are placing your body in jeopardy.*

All crash fad diets eliminate some important nutrients your body needs for optimal health. Although you can lose weight on these nutritionally unsound diets, you do so at the risk of your health and, in extreme diets, even your life. In addition, these unbalanced diets teach you bad eating habits which are difficult to get rid of later in life. They do not reeducate your taste buds—a curriculum vital to successful dieting and maintenance. It is true, that the majority of people who go on these diets do lose weight and do not get sick, because they do not stay on the diet long enough to cause their bodies real harm. But, since you don't know how long you can stay on an unbalanced diet safely, it is best that you avoid them altogether. After all, why should you play Russian Roulette with your health. What you want to do is to develop lifelong, sound eating habits, coupled with good exercise. It is impossible to do this on unbalanced diets.

Let's look first at three types of popular diets: Low-Protein Fad Diets, High-Protein Fad Diets, and High-Fat, Low-Carbohydrate Fad Diets. The last two are also called Ketogenic Diets.

LOW-PROTEIN FAD DIETS

Have all the nonprotein fruits and vegetables you want, limited carbohydrates and fats and no protein for several months. Eat no meat, poultry, fish, eggs, milk, cheese, nuts, or beans and peas that contain protein. This is what popular Low-Protein Fad Diets stipulate.

I contend that if you follow this advice you can harm your body. Not including protein in your diet throws your body into negative nitrogen balance, and it starts to break down or digest its own tissues. If you digest your heart you can have a heart attack. If you digest your kidneys you can develop kidney failure. If you digest your liver, you can develop liver disease. If you stayed on this diet long enough you would kill yourself. How you would die would depend on what part of your body, necessary for life, you were most readily absorbing. One eminent colleague told me he calculated that if you stayed on such a diet for 1,000 days you would quite simply disappear!

Since the next two diets are similar Ketogenic Diets, we describe each and then point out their defects.

HIGH-PROTEIN FAD DIETS

Drink large quantities of water a day and consume all the protein, including eggs, that you want. No carbohydrates and no fruits or vegetables allowed. On this diet you burn up 275 more calories than on a diet of the same number of calories that includes fruits, vegetables, and fats. When the body finds itself without carbohydrates for fuel, it begins burning its own body fat to supply energy. Stay on the diet until you're down to your ideal weight, or at least within five to fifteen pounds of it. Then go on a regular diet, eating anything, and simply counting calories for a few months, calling this a maintenance regimen. Then back to the High-Protein Fad Diet to burn off those last few pounds, and back again to the so-called maintenance regimen.

The designers of these eat-all-the-protein-you-want diets are supposedly protecting themselves by suggesting use of vitamin capsules. But we know that vitamins from food sources are more readily absorbed by your body than when taken in capsule form. You *need* sufficient carbohydrates in order to utilize the B complex vitamins.

Advocates of the High-Protein Fad Diets suggest you could

lose the most weight quickest by avoiding fruits and vegetables entirely. How dangerous and unsensible! Many fruits and vegetables are low in carbohydrates, and they are such excellent natural sources of vitamins and minerals. They also contain fiber and other roughage that help you have good elimination.

Let's get one thing straight: drinking even prodigious quantities of water will not make you lose weight. Neither will a combination of water and protein foods, per se. Certainly, water is a fine diuretic up to a point—it helps you get rid of excess fluid in and around your tissues. Equally important, water prevents you from becoming dehydrated; dehydration is excessive loss of body water, which excess water ingested prevents. And certainly, protein foods (meat, cheese, eggs) stay longer in your stomach and intestines before being digested and absorbed into the bloodstream. Therefore you have the feeling of being full for a longer period of time.

When you eat protein your metabolic rate increases and therefore you burn up more calories.

For every 130 calories of protein you take in you lose 30 automatically as body heat, so that you end up with 100.

For every 106 calories of fat, you lose 6 as heat; for every 104 calories of carbohydrates, you lose 4 as heat.

Providing you don't eat totally more calories than you burn up, this means you could eat about 25 percent more protein calories than carbohydrate or fat calories and not gain weight.

But the main reason a person loses weight on the High-Protein, Low-Carbohydrate Fad Diet is not because he up appreciably more calories, but because he eats less calories. You just can't eat as much heavy, harder-to-digest meat, eggs, and other protein as you can much easier-to-digest carbohydrates.

A case in point is Larry, a thirty-three year-old teacher,

who had a lesson to learn about losing weight. He was burning 2,831 calories a day and taking in 3,150. So the difference—319 calories a day, 2,233 calories a week—was consequently going to fat, and he was gaining 2¼ pounds a month. I examined him thoroughly and found there was nothing metabolically wrong with him. I gave him a 1,200 calorie, well-balanced diet. But he didn't go on it. Instead, on his own he went on a ketogenic diet for one month. His intake was now 1,650 calories a day. He was burning 3,000 calories a day. So he was losing 1,350 calories a day, or 9,450 calories a week—2¾ pounds a week. But his uric acid went up, he ran into a gout problem, and came back to see me. He then went on my 1,200 calorie balanced diet. He was now burning 2,916 calories, a difference of 1,716 calories a day—about 3 pounds a week.

"All right," you say, "so the High-Protein Fad Diets don't work because of the water or because of a magical water and protein combination. But they do work and they're easy to remember, although I admit they're a bore because they're so limited."

To which I must respond: I wish their worst feature were that they're boring. Boredom won't impair your health. In fact, *because* the diets are a bore, you tend to eat less and less of the protein as you go on with them, thereby taking in less calories. Providing your daily activity (energy expenditure) remains the same, the real reason why you're losing weight on these diets is that you are eating fewer calories.

But there are serious problems. A scientific study just concluded at an Eastern medical research center showed that normal people on these fad diets for only week increased their cholesterol levels. The researchers concluded that fad diets are potentially harmful to your health, especially for patients with any type of heart disease.

LOW-CARBOHYDRATE, HIGH-FAT FAD DIETS

Carbohydrates (which make up about 45 percent of most Americans' diets) are a no-no, advocates of these diets maintain. Many people, they theorize, including the over-weight, are unable to metabolize carbohydrate normally. Their formula: Eliminate carbohydrate altogether, so that your body is thrown into ketosis—the state in which ketone bodies, or acid chemicals, are formed. (More about ketosis later.) Then gradually restore a little carbohydrate, but not enough to stop the ketosis. Meanwhile eat all the fatty foods and protein you like.

What do the advocates of this diet say is happening? Your body has called forth a fat mobilizing hormone (FMH) manufactured by the pituitary gland. This is a thumbnail sketch of the formula which, I believe, is without scientific validity.

KETOGENIC DIETS

Q. What are the differences between these two main Ketogenic Diets?

A. One is a high-protein, low-carbohydrate diet served with lots of water. The other is a high-protein, low-carbohydrate diet served with lots of fat. From now on, both diets will be referred to as Ketogenic Diets.

Q. Are the Ketogenic Diets deficient in carbohydrates?

A. Yes, they are, therefore, the body burns up fat

defectively, producing ketone bodies. Ketone bodies are acid chemicals that result when fats are not completely broken down. This incomplete fat breakdown is what causes ketosis. Ketone bodies can make you feel less hungry because they depress the appetite center in the brain, *but this depression is done at the expense of possibly upsetting your body's delicate chemical balance.*

Advocates of these Ketogenic Diets want you to believe there is something magical about their specific diet that will cause you to lose weight. In reality the diets work simply because you are eating less calories than your body is burning. Ketogenic Diets operate on the principle that if you decrease your carbohydrate intake drastically, you cannot eat enough other foods to make up the calorie difference.

Ketogenic Diets cause the accumulation of *Ketone bodies* in your urine. These diets may cause the uric acid in your blood to increase and this, in susceptible people, can cause painful attacks of gout. Ketogenic Diets may do harm to the fetus of a pregnant mother. They could also be harmful to people with unsuspected kidney disease; they might retain urea. Such a diet in a person with an advanced state of kidney disease could promote kidney failure.

The first time I saw Ken, my eye was drawn to his right arm—to a tattoo of a lady who undulated seductively when he flexed his muscles. When Ken wasn't on the road driving a truck, he lived in Cincinnati. Recently his wife had remarked that he was spreading around the middle. This did not go with his image of his well-muscled body, so Ken decided to try a Ketogenic Diet. He had to carry a thermos around in the cab of his truck to get down large quantities of liquid a day. Until that time he had taken pride in his trouble-free body. On the diet, he forced himself to eat a great deal of protein. During the first week of dieting Ken lost three pounds, but on his tenth day his right big toe grew sore, red, and hot. It was so painful that he couldn't drive his truck. He stayed over in Pittsburgh to see a doctor who did a blood test. The doctor found he had a high uric acid level and gout and referred him to me. Ken was not previously aware that he had gout. The doctor told him the condition was aggravated by the diet and his body's incomplete breakdown of protein to uric acid. He was immediately taken off the diet and treated with proper medication for the gout. On my well-balanced diet, Ken has also lost his extra pounds.

Q. Can Ketogenic Diets cause extreme fatigue?

A. Two eminent researchers, W. F. Bloom and G. J. Azar, who published their work in medical literature, have reported that all the people they studied on carbohydrate-free diets complained of fatigue after two days on the diet:

"This complaint was characterized by a feeling of physical lack of energy and was brought on by physical activity. They all felt that they did not have sufficient energy to continue normal activity after the third day. This fatigue promptly disappeared after the addition of carbohydrate to the diet."

John was thirty-six and wore his black handlebar mustache well. His dress was casual though disheveled. He said he had been worrying about where his life as an auto worker was going. The same daily task, on the same plodding road, didn't seem to be leading in an upward direction as he had once hoped it would.

Eating became his substitute reward, until one evening his girlfriend grabbed the rolls around his middle and playfully christened them "love handles." At about the same time, he saw an ad promoting a Low-Carbohydrate, High-Fat Fad Diet. He went on it, and after five days, each time he got out of bed in the morning he got dizzy, as if the room were moving around him. When I examined him I found that when he got up from a prone position, his blood pressure dropped significantly—thus the sense of dizziness. This was probably a side effect of the diet. No medication was necessary. John was just taken off the diet and his dizziness stopped within seventy-two hours. I put him on our well-balanced diet and he is doing very well and losing weight. In their study, Bloom and Azar also observed this phenomenon. It is called "postural hypotension."

Q. Can a Ketogenic Diet cause constipation or diarrhea?
A. Yes, a Ketogenic Diet can lead to constipation and, if you have a concomitant medical problem, it can lead to diarrhea as illustrated by Pam's case, below.

On a Ketogenic Diet you can have problems because of the inadequacy of green, leafy vegetables. You *need* these vegetables to provide roughage so as to avoid hard, painful stools. And if you don't absorb foods properly and don't get enough vitamin A for many months, you can also have problems with mucous membranes, eyes, and skin. Lack of vitamin A can lower your resistance to infection.

When I first examined Pam, her pretty blue eyes were rimmed with red, dry, and itchy lids. Although she had not had trouble with her skin since adolescence, now, at thirty-eight, she noticed it was excessively dry and flaky in spite of the creams and lotions she hopefully rubbed in nightly. She had also developed more colds than usual.

Pam was a real estate agent in Jackson, Mississippi. In the process of showing houses she had overheard an unkind remark from a prospective buyer who was following her up the stairs from the basement. She was fifteen pounds overweight, and from that moment painfully aware of it. In six months her daughter was graduating from high school. Pam wanted to have an open house for the family and friends, so she set a target date for weight loss that didn't give her much leeway. She badly wanted to be thinner.

She put herself on a Ketogenic Diet, then felt "rotten." After four months on a self-imposed vitamin-A deficient diet and because of persistent diarrhea, she came to me with all her symptoms and was even more frantic to lose weight. A series of tests were performed and Pam was found not to be absorbing fats properly, thus causing the diarrhea, and deficient in vitamin A. The diet was partially to blame. She was treated with proper enzymes, diet, and given adequate amounts of vitamin A. Within three months she lost her fifteen pounds; her skin and eye problems cleared; she no longer had a low resistance to infection. And she no longer needed vitamin A, since she got it in her diet by eating such foods as carrots, liver, and green leafy vegetables. Diet and enzymes have controlled her diarrhea.

Q. Can ketones hurt the unborn fetus of a pregnant woman?
A. A study sponsored by the National Institute of Neurological Diseases and Stroke showed that children of women with acetone (a ketone) in their urine during pregnancy were significantly less intelligent than those of comparable mothers without this metabolic imbalance. Ketone bodies can also cause damage to the brain of the unborn fetus.

Q. Could a child be born mentally retarded because of these ketone bodies?
A. The possibility, *though remote*, does exist. Therefore, I would especially urge pregnant women to shun these potentially hazardous diets.

*As I tell my private patients, notwithstanding what they
hear from the faddists, I advocate a nutritionally sound
diet for all people, but especially for pregnant mothers.
Because of possible harm to the fetus, women should not
restrict nutrients lower than their body needs during
pregnancy.*

Q. **Has the United States Congress become aware of the fad
diets Americans are being encouraged to try?**
A. Yes. The Select Committee on Nutrition and Human
Needs of the United States Senate has begun holding
hearings on obesity and fad diets.

At those hearings, the American Medical Association
came out loud and clear against fad diets. They
particularly pointed out that Ketogenic Diets, because of
their unlimited intake of saturated fats and cholesterol-
rich foods could promote blood clots and heart problems.

That's how I happened to meet Joe. As Joe got older,
year by year the pounds crept up. He rarely exercised or
walked, except for going to and from his car. By the age of
sixty-two he was a fat, balding, successful plastics
manufacturer, fifty-two pounds too heavy, but with a
history of good health. One night while sitting in his
Boston living room, he heard about a Ketogenic Diet on
one of the television talk shows. The idea that he could eat
fatty food, yet still lose weight, appealed to Joe. He loved
fatty foods, but his family doctor had strictly cautioned
him against them, so he had always monitored his fat
intake carefully. That was wise, because Joe had a family
history of heart disease. He was elated to hear he could
have all the eggs, pork, bacon, and ham he wanted, even
every day. Joe had been limiting these foods for so long
that he began to eat "retroactively"—satisfying his past
cravings. All he ate was fatty foods, day in and day out.

After five months he experienced severe pain in his left leg. He went to his family doctor, who found Joe had developed a clot in a blood vessel in his left leg. Joe also experienced chest pains whenever he walked any distance. After taking appropriate tests, including an electrocardiogram, his doctor confirmed he had developed a heart problem. He explained that the high fat and cholesterol content in Joe's blood possibly resulting from the diet could have caused the blood vessel to clot, and the heart problem. Joe was taken off the Ketogenic Diet, given blood thinner, and referred to me. I put him on my well-balanced, low-cholesterol, low-calorie diet. After three months of treatment he was back to work, feeling good, and thirty-three pounds trimmer.

In people like Joe, who respond to a low-carbohydrate, high fatty food diet with a high rise of fat in their blood, the risk of coronary artery disease and other signs of hardening of the arteries may well be increased—particularly if the diet is maintained over a prolonged period. Some of these signs and symptoms may be chest pain, irregular electrocardiogram, palpitations, and pain radiating down the arms, all early warning signs of a possible heart attack.

Another patient referred to me because of heart problems probably related to his bad diet was William, a fifty-seven year-old gray-haired railroad man from Erie, Pennsylvania. He had been told by one of his passengers that by going on a Ketogenic Diet he could eat all the eggs he wanted. William's family doctor had previously warned him against eating more than three eggs a week because of a cholesterol and triglyceride (fat) problem. Without the advice of his doctor, William went on the fad diet, and after three months he developed a fluttering feeling in his chest. He went back to his doctor, who took an electrocardiogram and blood tests. The electrocardiogram revealed that he had arrhythmia and atherosclerosis (increased accumulation of fatty deposits on the inside of his arteries). His doctor took him off the high-cholesterol diet and referred him to me. I put him on a low-cholesterol diet and medication to lower his cholesterol. On this regimen William has done very well. His cholesterol has dropped from 450 to a normal 175. His heart now has a normal rhythm. To help keep his cholesterol in check, William only eats one egg a week. He has now lost thirty-four pounds as a result of reducing calories.

Q. **Ketogenic Diets allow excessive amounts of protein. Can this be harmful?**

A. Devastating medical harm could come to a person with an unsuspected kidney problem that results in nitrogen retention. Such a person, consuming this excess protein, could increase his blood urea nitrogen until he becomes poisoned with urea, unconscious, and even near death. *No one should go on any type of diet without first consulting a physician.* This applies even before embarking on a nutritionally balanced diet, i.e., one that includes adequate daily amounts of nutrients (carbohydrates, fats, proteins) and micronutrients (vitamins and minerals).

Fred came to me after a costly, harrowing experience. At twenty-six, he had a medium build with brown hair and eyes to match. He was a pleasant fellow, not terribly overweight—about fifteen pounds. He lived in Denver and worked in a chemical factory. During years of work he had breathed a tremendous amount of mercury vapor. Fred developed unsuspected kidney disease, probably triggered by the mercury in his system. Not knowing this, when he had put on so many extra pounds that his pants started getting hard to close, he decided to try a Ketogenic Diet he had heard about on television. After two months on the diet he became very bloated and had a strange urinelike odor to his breath. Because he felt so tired, and because his wife objected to his bad breath, he went to his doctor, who did a blood test and a SUN (serum urea nitrogen—a test to determine how much urea nitrogen is in the blood). This showed he had an increased amount of urea in his blood. He was hospitalized and put on an artificial kidney machine to take the poisons out of his blood.

His doctor told him the reason he had the high urea was because of poor kidney function aggravated by too much protein in the diet. It was indeed fortunate that he saw his doctor, because otherwise he could have lapsed into coma and even death.

After his frightening experience, Fred still wanted to lose his excess pounds, but sanely. I put him on my diet, modified for kidney disease, and suggested he change jobs. On this regimen he has done exceptionally well, losing the fifteen pounds in seven and a half weeks. He is also under the care of a kidney specialist, who, incidently, found him a hospital job as an orderly—a job which includes reading the mercury on thermometers and blood pressure instruments.

Q. **Some advocates of Ketogenic Diets say there is no problem with vitamin deficiencies, yet they tell you to take not just ordinary doses, but extra large doses called megavitamins. Is this a good idea?**

A. No, you don't need massive amounts of vitamins (megavitamins). Fortunately the Food and Drug Administration has made it supremely difficult for you to poison your body with large doses of vitamins A and D. The FDA maintains that excessive amounts of vitamin A taken over long periods can increase pressure within the human skull. This pressure may appear to be a brain tumor. Vitamins A and D in excessive dosages, the FDA said, can retard mental and physical growth in children. Sale of vitamin A is now restricted to 10,000 units, and vitamin D to 400 units.

However, anyone who chooses to go on a Ketogenic Diet will need some vitamin supplementation. Also if you know you are not taking the time to eat properly, then you may well be shortchanging your body of its vitamin and mineral requirements. You can have your blood tested to see what nutrients you are deficient in, and then take the appropriate vitamin and mineral supplements prescribed by your doctor. Your physician probably will not suggest such a blood test to you; you will probably have to ask him for one that specifically measures your blood vitamins and minerals. He may not do the procedure, but he can find a lab for you that does it.

Do not overdose yourself on vitamins. You should not put anything in your body it does not need, including large doses of megavitamins. Too many vitamins can cause serious problems, just as a lack of vitamins can.

Unfortunately, you cannot find on the market today a single pill or capsule that contains exactly 100 percent of the recommended dietary allowance (RDA) for the vitamins and minerals your body needs.

As an intern at the Johns Hopkins Hospital, I began researching the world's medical and nutritional literature for all the best scientific data available on the body's many vitamin and mineral needs. I developed the following dietary supplement, called cofactrol, for each stage of life and presented it to the Food and Drug Administration. The FDA concurred that each supplement is exactly 100 percent of the recommended dietary allowance of all known vitamins and minerals for each group. My formula is identical to the new (1974) Recommended Dietary Allowances formulated by the National Research Council.

The supplement is not now available on the market. Nobody makes one capsule or wafer that supplies exactly 100 percent of your daily need of all known nutrients. Private industry should certainly do so, but no company has. Instead, the market is flooded with many different bottles of single or multiple vitamins—some with, some without, minerals—usually in much more than the 100 percent that you need. If you were trying to buy a complete dietary supplement today, you couldn't find it unless you took bits and pieces of many different pills and capsules, and then it would cost you plenty.

THE FOLLOWING IS EXACTLY 100 PERCENT OF THE RDA OF EACH VITAMIN AND MINERAL FOR EACH OF 4 GROUPS:

VAM (or vitamins and minerals) for infants from birth until 12 months of age

VAM for children over one but under four years of age

1,500 IU (international units) vitamin A	2,500 IU vitamin A
400 IU vitamin D	400 IU vitamin D
5.0 IU vitamin E	10 IU vitamin E
35 mg ascorbic acid (vitamin C)	40 mg ascorbic acid (vitamin C)
0.5 mg thiamin (vitamin B1)	0.7 mg thiamin (vitamin B1)
0.6 mg riboflavin (vitamin B2)	0.8 mg riboflavin (vitamin B2)
	9.0 mg niacin

8.0 mg niacin
0.4 mg vitamin B₆
0.1 mg folic acid
2.0 mcg vitamin B₁₂
0.05 mg biotin
3.0 mg pantothenic acid
0.6 gm calcium
0.5 gm phosphorus
15 mg iron
45 mcg iodine
5.0 mg zinc
70 mg magnesium
0.6 mg copper

0.7 mg vitamin B₆
0.2 mg folic acid
3.0 mcg vitamin B₁₂
0.15 mg biotin
5.0 mg pantothenic acid
0.8 gm calcium
0.8 gm phosphorus
10 mg iron
70 mcg iodine
8.0 mg zinc
200 mg magnesium
1.0 mg copper

VAM for adults and children four or more years

VAM for use in pregnant or lactating women

5,000 IU vitamin A
400 IU vitamin D
30 IU vitamin E
60 mg ascorbic acid (vitamin C)
1.5 mg thiamin (vitamin B₁)
1.7 mg riboflavin (vitamin B₂)
20 mg niacin
2.0 mg vitamin B₆
0.4 mg folic acid
6.0 mcg vitamin B₁₂
0.3 mg biotin
10 mg pantothenic acid
1.0 g calcium
1.0 g phosphorus
18 mg iron
150 mcg iodine
15 mg zinc
400 mg magnesium
2.0 mg copper

8,000 IU vitamin A
400 IU vitamin D
30 IU vitamin E
60 mg ascorbic acid (vitamin C)
1.7 mg thiamin (vitamin B₁)
2.0 mg riboflavin (vitamin B₂)
20 mg niacin
2.5 mg vitamin B₆
0.8 mg folic acid
8.0 mcg vitamin B₁₂
0.3 mg biotin
10 mg pantothenic acid
1.3 gm calcium
1.3 gm phosphorus
18 mg iron
150 mcg iodine
15 mg zinc
450 mg magnesium
2.0 mg copper

I have also given the VAM formula to the Department of Agriculture, which could efficiently dispense it to children with school lunches. And I have given it to the Department of Health, Education and Welfare in the hope that it may see fit to give the supplement to poor people in order to prevent vitamin and mineral deficiencies.

Remember—you should not take vitamin pills indiscriminately. You will urinate much of the excess vitamins—your money will literally go down the drain! If you eat a normal, well-balanced diet, you probably don't need additional vitamins. You don't have to guess. Your doctor can have your blood tested to see if you are deficient in any one vitamin or mineral.

Q. Advocates of the Ketogenic Diets maintain you don't have to worry about a deficiency of carbohydrates because fat can be converted to carbohydrates in sufficient amounts. What about that?

A. They are wrong again. Their statement is just plain biochemically incorrect, and there is scientific data to disprove it.

When Fran came to see me, I could tell she was only about ten pounds overweight, all carried in her hips and thighs. She was slightly built, short and pretty in her mid-forties. Her hair was a mass of well-coiffed dark brown curls piled high on her head. She said it made her feel taller and drew attention from the problem-area waist downward. She lived in Beaumont, Texas, and worked there for the power company.

One day while waiting in her dentist's office, she picked up a woman's magazine featuring a Ketogenic Diet. She had only nine pounds to lose—the sooner the better—so she went all out on it. Little did she know she was susceptible to the dangers of a low-carbohydrate diet. After being on the diet for only one day she became nauseated. On the second day she started vomiting and was so fatigued she couldn't go to work. As the day wore on she became progressively more listless. The third day her roommate noticed that her face was drawn, her eyes were sunken, and her breath had a fruity odor. Alarmed, she called her local doctor. He took one look at Fran and told her she was suffering from dehydration because of the low-carbohydrate diet. He admitted her to the hospital's emergency ward where he gave her intravenous fluid. Fran did well on this regimen and was released after thirty-six hours with directions for a well-balanced diet. When she had been built up again, her doctor sent her to me. She is now on my nutritionally sound reducing diet, is losing her nine pounds, and her hazel eyes have regained their shine. Along with the diet, I have prescribed exercises to tone the hips and thighs. Fran's experience, although rare, was similar to that recorded by the Canadian Army Study during World War II, in which performance of soldiers rapidly deteriorated and they became seriously ill from loss of needed body fluid associated with carbohydrate-free diets.

Q. **What is the true relationship between hypoglycemia (low blood sugar) and obesity?**

A. The AMA Council reported: "Recent publicity in the popular press has led the public to believe that the occurrence of hypoglycemia is widespread in this country. . . . These claims are not supported by medical evidence. Because of the possible misunderstanding about the matter, three organizations of physicians and scientists (The American Diabetes Association, the Endocrine Society, and the American Medical Association) have spelled out the signs of hypoglycemia. 'Hypoglycemia means a low level of blood sugar. When it occurs, it is often attended by symptoms of sweating, shakiness, trembling, anxiety, fast heart action, headache, hunger sensations, brief feelings of weakness, and, occasionally, seizures and coma.' "

Mary is a striking woman with green eyes and bright orange hair. She lives in Des Moines. For fourteen of her thirty-two years she has worked in a wholesale house. For the past four years, she had had an undiagnosed illness that kept her miserable. After eating sweets, Mary would develop sweating, shakiness, trembling, and often a feeling of anxiety. On many occasions after eating candy, Mary's heart would race and she would become headachy.

On other occasions, after eating cake she would become hungry, then develop a sense of weakness. She had been to several doctors who told her it was a functional problem in her mind—that there was nothing organically wrong with her. While she was visiting friends in Baltimore, they couldn't help noticing how mercurial she had become; how irritable and shaky. They were concerned, and convinced her to be worked up at Johns Hopkins Hospital, where she had a battery of tests including a glucose tolerance test. The results were abnormal. Her blood sugar shot up, then immediately fell to below normal levels. The tests revealed she was what I term a "carboholic" (in other words, she could not handle carbohydrates properly, a mild form of low blood sugar). I put her on my Easy, No-Risk Diet for carboholics (see Chapter 4), and after two months of painless dieting she continues to do exceptionally well, having lost eleven pounds, and no longer showing any of the symptoms. Our special diet provides adequate but not excessive carbohydrates. It is well balanced and contains all the nutrients your body needs.

Do not indulge in self-diagnosis. It is important to remember what the three medical societies go on to point out: "However, the majority of people with these kinds of symptoms do not have hypoglycemia. A great many patients with anxiety reactions have similar symptoms. Furthermore, there is no good evidence that hypoglycemia causes depression, chronic fatigue, allergies, nervous breakdowns, alcoholism, juvenile delinquency, childhood behavior problems, drug addiction, or inadequate sexual performance. . . ."

My esteemed colleague, Dr. Philip L. White, Secretary of the AMA's Council on Food and Nutrition, writing against fad diets in the American Medical Association magazine, *Today's Health,* said Ketogenic Diets can be unhealthy because they are deficient in carbohydrate. Writes Dr. White: "The National Research Council suggests that persons accustomed to normal diets need at least 100 grams of carbohydrates per day to avoid ketosis, excessive protein breakdown and other undesirable metabolic responses." Some Ketogenic Diets start with zero carbohydrates and go up to a maximum of 50 grams of carbohydrates a day. Since 30 grams approximates one ounce, you are taking in about one half the amount of carbohydrates a normal body needs every day.

Q. Can't the body convert protein to sugar if you don't have enough sugar in your diet?

A. Fortunately the body has a mechanism, known as gluconeogenesis. This converts protein to sugar. If, however, you have an endocrine gland imbalance of which you are not aware, you might indeed be courting trouble by going on such a diet. What's more, no two human bodies have identical rates of converting protein into sugar. Therefore, how can you know whether your conversion rate is adequate to ward off problems?

Q. How did these fad diets become so popular?

A. The popularity of fad dieting has its origin with the Zen Buddhist Macrobiotic Diet. That, or one of its variants, of all the bad diets, has caused the most people to become sick and even die from malnutrition.

The original diet regimen prescribed eating only natural cereals three times a day, a small amount of water, and gomasio, which is four parts seasoned seed sprinkled with one part sea salt. The diet lacks B vitamins as well as adequate protein. It should be called the microbiotic (tendency to decrease life) rather than macrobiotic (tendency to prolong life) diet.

Many parents are properly concerned about the possible muscle and nerve damage that can result if their child stays on a diet that is 100 percent vegetarian. Any such diet must lack vitamin B_{12}, which is necessary for normal nerve and muscle function. Such children often have problems walking because of the deficiency of B_{12}. If you feel that you or your child must go on a vegetarian diet, then add eggs, milk, soybean products, and/or fish to get adequate B_{12}. If necessary, your doctor could prescribe B_{12} for you.

There is still another popular group of fad diets that promises you the impossible—to eat all you want and still lose weight. Every few years an allegedly new and magic diet sweeps our too-often gullible land. Many of these, as previously discussed, are high-protein, low-carbohydrate diets based on the fallacious theory that protein won't cause you to gain weight. Nonsense! Any food can make you fat if you eat too much of it. A calorie is a calorie is a calorie! For every gram of protein you eat, you take in four calories; for every gram of carbohydrate you eat, you take in the same number—four. A gram of fat yields nine calories. And calories *do* count—every time, all the time. If you are overweight, you are taking in more calories than your body needs, and the excess is being turned into fat.

To lose weight you must take in fewer calories than your body needs so that fat will be burned up to meet energy requirements.

Your weight reflects the number of calories you take in, minus the number of calories you burn. As I said before, it is true that you do burn up more calories in eating a gram of protein than a gram of carbohydrate. *But the reason you lose significant weight on any diet is simply because you eat less.* In other words you take in less food which means you take in less calories.

Q. Where did the other crash fad diets originate? What happened to them?

A. The majority are no more than low-carbohydrate, high-protein diets, or, as previously called, Ketogenic Diets. Each has its own unbalanced gimmick. Before coming to me, many of my patients had tried them.

One fad diet you should avoid is the no-fat 500-calorie diet you eat every day while your doctor injects you with urine—not just regular urine, but special urine from pregnant women. The program consists of the daily injection of HCG (human chorionic gonadotrophin) containing this urine and depends on your staying on a 500-calorie fat-free diet.

The case that best exemplifies my lack of faith in HCG involves identical twins, John and William, age eighteen, from Philadelphia. Both weighed 200 pounds, were 5 feet 9 inches, and had blue eyes and brown hair. Both had the same type of small bone structure and both found they felt and functioned best at an ideal weight of 147 pounds.

John went to a doctor who administered the shots from a pregnant woman's urine. He went daily for the injections and stuck to the 500-calorie diet. William went to their family doctor. William told him about John's receiving the shots, and the family doctor put him on the identical diet but gave him daily shots of what were nothing but plain unadulterated water (no urine). But William thought he was getting the same urine shots as John. Both stayed on a 500-calorie no-fat diet.

At the end of one month, John, who had gone for the daily urine shots, lost twenty-two pounds and claimed he had no problem staying on the diet. William, on exactly the same diet, but receiving a water placebo instead of the urine shot, lost twenty-one pounds but did have difficulty staying on the diet. He was hungry most of the time.

The conclusion is that the urine shots really didn't matter all that much. It was mainly the diet of only 500 calories and the daily reinforcement of seeing their doctor that allowed the twins, and allows you, to lose weight. The cost of John's urine shots for the month was $260. The cost of William's visits to his doctor for the month was $25. It was a considerable difference in the cost to each if not in the weight they lost.

I had a chance to study John and William in Baltimore after they had been on the diet for one month. At that time, John weighed 178 pounds and William 179 pounds. A test to determine how many calories they actually burned was performed. This is a very simple test in which you lie down on a table, face up. The amount of oxygen you breath in and the amount of carbon dioxide you breathe out is measured. From this I determine what is called the respiratory quotient, RQ, which tells you how many calories and what percent fat, carbohydrate, and protein your body burns. John and William each burned 3,000 calories a day. Since the diet they had been on previously was a 500-calorie diet, that means that they were in negative calorie balance of 2,500 calories a day. On seven days a week they were in negative balance of 17,500 calories. You burn one pound of fat for every 3,500 calories that you burn, above what you take in. Since they had burned 17,500 calories more than they had taken in, they each lost at the rate of 5 pounds a week. Therefore, *any* diet they could have been on which would have only allowed them 500 calories a day would have resulted in this same weight loss. They then went on my 1,200-calorie easy, no-risk diet and each of them found it much easier to tolerate and lost at the rate of 5 pounds a month until each reached his ideal weight of 147 pounds.

They are now on my Figure-Keeper maintenance regimen and are able to maintain their ideal weight.

The unfortunate part about this is that many fat people go on a 500-calorie diet while not under a doctor's supervision. They can become very weak and encounter serious medical problems.

I had spoken to the late Dr. A. T. W. Simeons, who was the first to use HCG in the treatment of human obesity, and he guaranteed me that he envisioned no one going on the 500-calorie diet who was not under the constant, careful scrutiny of a doctor. Before subjecting yourself and your pocketbook to this treatment, I would first recommend getting counsel and advice from your family doctor.

Other unbalanced diets, all of which should be avoided, have been popularized in magazines. The Grapefruit Diet was developed by *Harper's Bazaar* in 1941. Mary, a Houston housewife who went on a modified grapefruit diet in 1961, told me when I took her history and examined her as an intern: "If you eat a half grapefruit before each meal, you just don't want too much during the meal." She ate 800 calories a day on the Grapefruit Diet.

The Snack Diet—another variant of the low-carbohydrate, high-protein diet—was brought to the public's attention by *McCall's* in 1970. It called for snacking all day rather than eating three square meals. "Most of my fat customers only eat one meal a day—but it lasts all day long," said Barbara, a Los Angeles model for fat women's clothes. On the Snack Diet, Barbara was eating 860 calories a day. When I tested her I found her body was burning 1,480 calories a day, so she would have lost weight on any diet less than 1,480 calories.

Vogue in 1964 called for six meals a day—morning, midmorning, noon, midafternoon, early evening, and late evening—and called it the Nibbling Diet. Betty Jo, a waitress from Seattle, said: "Before going on this diet I was always stuffing my face in between times. I felt awfully guilty but I just couldn't help myself. Then I read about the Nibbling Diet and now I eat more than my three meals a day—I nibble six times a day—but I no longer feel guilty about it." The Nibbling Diet gave her 1,000 calories a day. When I tested Betty Jo, I found she was burning 1,835 calories a day. That is why she was losing weight on the Nibbling Diet.

The No-Hunger Rice Diet published by *Coronet* in 1960 was a takeoff of Dr. Walter Kempner's Rice Diet developed thirty years ago. This variation combined Chinese and American style cooking with the net result being a decreased number of calories going into the mouth. This was the diet elected by Mao Woo, a San Francisco restaurateur, who said: "Fat Orientals, like fat old people, are hard to find." He took in 950 calories a day. When I tested him, he was burning 2,633 calories a day.

Look in 1963 popularized the Hot Dog Diet. This diet permitted you to have three pure beef frankfurters a day, each wrapped in a piece of bread, plus condiments and some vegetables. To Shirley, a student from Columbus, Ohio, this was like being on a prolonged picnic. She ate 900 calories per day and burned up 1,703 calories a day.

Plato was the father of the vegetarian diet now commonly called the Vegetable and Fruit Diet, which has had Gandhi, George Bernard Shaw, and Nehru as its exponents. Eating only fruits and vegetables wouldn't be a safe way to reduce. Fruits and vegetables do not contain vitamin B_{12}. It is in eggs and meats, and necessary for healthy nerve and muscle function—particularly in children.

The Milk Diet originated a century ago, but in 1954 it was modified and became known as the Rockefeller Diet. The original diet allowed for no solid foods—only liquids for four meals a day. Don, a radio announcer from Philadelphia, remembers the diet well, for "it was the only diet I tried where I didn't require a laxative." He was sipping 900 calories a day, while burning 3,004 calories a day.

The Meat and Mushroom Diet got its push from *Look* in 1962. You ate nine ounces of meat and twenty fresh mushrooms a day. Surprisingly, Paul, a garage mechanic in Jersey City, said: "If I could afford it today and hadn't become dizzy on the diet, I'd be back on it." When I examined him I found his dizziness resulted from an inadequate supply of micronutrients (vitamins and minerals). Obviously his 700 calories a day were not enough for him. He burned 2,672 calories a day.

The Skim Milk and Banana Diet originated from Pittsburgh's Highland Park Zoo area thirty-five years ago: three 8-ounce glasses of skim milk a day along with a banana. Chester, a porter at the Chicago Zoo, thought it a great diet for monkeys; nevertheless, he stayed on it for three weeks and was only getting 625 calories a day. When I tested him I found he was burning 2,777 calories daily.

In 1964 *Vogue* popularized the Egg and Wine Diet. You ate five eggs a day and killed a twenty-four-ounce bottle of wine along with them. You felt no pain but your cholesterol rose and your liver was endangered. As Tom, one of New York's finest, said:"Some people will try anything." Before he was discharged from the Police Force and drinking more than one bottle of wine a day, he was consuming 1,200 calories daily. I tested him and found he was burning 2,999 calories.

"Diet! Start Losing!" Cottage Cheese Blintz Diet limits your daily calorie intake to about 500. Donna, a waitress from Phoenix, complained: "After ten days on this diet you actually start feeling like cottage cheese." When I tested Donna I found she was burning 1,227 calories a day.

The Saturday Evening Post popularized the Steak and Tomato Diet about 1942. It called for a steak and a medium-sized tomato at every meal, and if hungry, a tomato at bedtime. It was worth 700 calories a day, and Ted, a sports car racer from Indianapolis, felt: "If you can afford it, it's great—that is, for a while." Ted was burning 2,631 calories daily.

The Egg and Orange Diet originated in France and hit the United States in 1950. Its mainstay was three eggs and two and a half oranges a day. It added up to about 550 calories and, to quote Virginia, a school teacher from Trenton, "It doesn't require any gourmet cooking." She was burning 1,481 calories a day.

The Strawberry and Cream Diet was pushed by *Woman's Home Companion* and consisted of eating five cups of strawberries topped with eight tablespoons of sour cream every day. You get about 550 calories this way, and it appealed to Betty Joe, a Detroit salesgirl, who thought: "It might not be nutritionally sound, but it sure tastes good." She was burning 1,809 calories.

The most recent of the crash, fad diets is the Pumpkin-Carrot Diet now sweeping Australia. You eat half a pumpkin and ten carrots a day. You take in less than 600 calories, but there is one major problem—it didn't take Cynthia, a bank teller from Melbourne, long to notice. "After two weeks on the diet my skin turned yellowish-orange." Her gynecologist reported that the ovaries of many women who went on the diet turned orange, there were a lot of irregular periods, and a number of women were unnecessarily concerned about being pregnant.

A recent fad promises that you can eat away fat deposits from your stomach, thighs, hips, and buttocks by avoiding certain "polluting" foods. The proponents give a list of foods to avoid that is totally unscientific. Worse, the limits put on meat, fish, and poultry—no more than once a day or every other day—can lead to protein deficiency and lack of iron. This can make you feel tired and irritable. The only way you can lose fat selectively from a part of your body is to go on a nutritionally sound diet and specifically exercise that part of your body where you want to spot reduce.

On the other hand the Amazing Cider Vinegar, Lecithin, Kelp, B6 Diet which appeared recently in *Family Circle* magazine is just as unbalanced. The author does mention that large amounts of vinegar are hard on your teeth, and that's the only thing we agree upon. Imagine eating kelp, B6, Lecithin and vinegar: You can get too much iodine from eating too much kelp. Too much iodine can turn off your normally functioning thyroid gland and cause you to have a sluggish thyroid. Then you will really gain weight, feel tired, and be listless. It would be wonderful if Lecithin would emulsify fat in the spots desired. But if this were fact—if one kept eating Lecithin—one would simply become a bottle of salad oil.

But the most bizarre of all these diet regimens is the Teeth Clamped Diet. Although it is successful from the point of view of losing weight, it certainly is not a viable way to keep weight off permanently.

Charles Smith, a thirty-two-year-old English male nurse, a bachelor, weighed 322 pounds. He had a heavy appetite, each day eating a whole chicken, four sandwiches, a pound of beef, gobs of potatoes, a dozen slices of toast, cookies, a pound of chocolate, and quarts of sweetened tea and coffee. Because his doctor felt there was no way to keep him from eating large amounts of food, short of clamping his mouth shut, this was indeed done. The clamp was installed by a dental surgeon, who described it as similar to clamps that are used for setting broken jaws. Charles' mouth was bolted shut, so that all he could do was sip liquids. He was on this regimen for 112 days. He mainly sipped milk and lost 105 pounds. He had a fifty-inch waist before he had his mouth clamped shut; a thirty-eight-inch waist afterward.

Mrs. Shirley Turner of Nottingham, England, was sixty-nine pounds lighter after four months of having her jaws cemented together with the insertion of a silver plate by her surgeon. She is down from 247 to 178 pounds and plans to keep her mouth shut till she has sipped her way to her bikini size of 133 pounds. A recent issue of *People* magazine cited other cases of diet by dental clamping. But I really cannot recommend mouth cement or a mouth clamp for lasting weight loss.

With the rapid proliferation of fad diets and their seductive promises of virtual overnight victory over weight problems—*and their corollary risks to your health*—it is all the more important that you find and embrace a nutritionally sound, safe, and balanced diet that will allow you to develop a lifetime pattern of good, health-giving eating habits, as well as adequate exercise. The Easy, No-Risk Diet offers that opportunity. But first, you must determine your ideal weight.

2

FIRST
DETERMINE
YOUR IDEAL
WEIGHT

Are you tired? Are you tired of being fat? Tired of dieting? Tired of being a yo-yo—of going to all the effort of losing weight and then finding that it suddenly comes right back? Are you disgusted with the whole bit? I don't blame you if you are. But do you want to try it one more time—make one final effort? *And do it without risk to your health?* If so, I can help you.

We are going to start by determining your goal. That is your *ideal* weight. The weight at which you will feel best. The weight at which you will look best. It's easy. All you need is a tape measure and my ideal weight table found on the next pages. Once you have determined your best weight it becomes your goal. Everything you do will be directed at achieving and staying at your ideal weight. Following my Easy, No-Risk Diet in the next chapter will lead you successfully to your goal. Then, to remain slim, simply follow my easy Figure-Keeper Maintenance Diet. This will allow you to stay at your ideal weight throughout your life.

So if you are serious about attaining your ideal weight and staying there once and for all, this book can give you the simple tools to achieve it; tools I have developed after seeing over 1,000 patients with weight problems. It's not difficult. It asks nothing of you beyond scrupulously following my directions.

As a result of carefully determining the ideal weights of these patients I have constructed the following table:

FOR MEN
IDEAL WEIGHT RANGE IN POUNDS
Age—18 Years and Over

Height Without Shoes	Small-Boned Range	Medium-Boned Range	Large-Boned Range
5'0"	100–120	103–127	108–132
5'1"	103–127	108–132	112–138
5'2"	109–133	113–139	118–144
5'3"	113–139	118–144	122–150
5'4"	119–145	123–151	128–156
5'5"	121–151	128–156	132–162
5'6"	125–157	133–163	138–168
5'7"	129–163	138–168	142–174
5'8"	133–169	143–175	148–180
5'9"	137–175	147–180	152–186
5'10"	141–182	151–187	157–193
5'11"	145–187	155–193	162–198
6'0"	150–194	159–199	166–205
6'1"	160–199	165–205	170–210
6'2"	168–206	173–211	177–217
6'3"	173–211	177–217	182–222
6'4"	178–218	183–223	187–229
6'5"	183–223	187–229	192–234
6'6"	188–230	193–235	197–241
6'7"	193–235	197–241	202–246

FOR WOMEN
IDEAL WEIGHT RANGE IN POUNDS
Age—18 Years and Older

Height Without Shoes	Small-Boned Range	Medium-Boned Range	Large-Boned Range
4'8"	85– 95	92–102	97–117
4'9"	87– 98	94–105	99–120
4'10"	89–101	96–108	101–123
4'11"	91–104	98–111*	104–126
5'0"	92–110	99–116	105–121
5'1"	94–116	100–121	106–127
5'2"	99–121	103–127	108–132
5'3"	103–127	108–132	112–138
5'4"	108–132	112–138	117–143
5'5"	112–138	117–143	121–149
5'6"	117–143	121–149	126–154
5'7"	121–149	126–154	130–160
5'8"	126–154	130–160	135–165
5'9"	130–160	135–165	139–171
5'10"	135–165	139–171	144–176
5'11"	139–171	144–176	148–182
6'0"	144–176	148–182	153–187
6'1"	149–181	153–186	158–193
6'2"	154–186	158–192	163–199

To determine your ideal weight you need first to know your exact height, without shoes. If you don't know how tall you are, stand against a flat surface looking forward, with both feet flat on the floor and your buttocks and the back of your head against the surface, such as a wall or door. Then have someone place a pencil flat on the top of your head and draw a small line. Measure the distance from the bottom of the floor to the line. This is your height.

Next you must determine if you have small, medium, or large bones. If you don't know your bone structure, you should ask the next time you see your doctor. As a rule of thumb, though, if you have delicate features, you have a small bone structure. If you have heavy features, you have a large bone structure. If you are like the majority of people, in between, then you have a medium bone structure.

A simple way to determine your bone size is to measure your wrist. Take a tape measure and measure around your wrist at the point of the two bumps. Women: If you measure anything under 6 inches, you have a small-boned frame. If you measure between 6 to 6½ inches, you have a medium-boned frame, and if you measure over 6½ inches, you have a large-boned frame. Men: Under 6 inches is small; 6–7 inches is medium; anything over 7 inches is large. Men and women measure both wrists. If the measurement is different for the two wrists, add the total and divide by two. If you have ever broken one wrist, just use the unbroken one.

It is possible to have small wrists but medium-sized bones elsewhere. Your doctor can advise you. Ten percent of my patients' wristbone sizes differed from the proportion of some other bones in their body, a variance taken into consideration in the Table's range of weight for each height and body frame.

Dr. C. Wesley Dupertuis, Professor of Clinical Anthropology at Case Western Reserve University School of Medicine, has done outstanding in-depth research in this area. He was my teacher when I was a young medical student at Case Western Reserve, and I have always had the utmost respect for him and his work. From his data I constructed the following table.

Parts of the Body	Percent of Total Body Weight
Head	8%
Arms	12%
Upper body trunk	23%
Lower body trunk	24%
Legs	33%

He also found that your wrist size is a good approximation of whether you are small, medium, or large boned compared to your height.

Q. How do I know my best weight within the range in your table?
A. It is the weight within your range at which you feel best.

Q. Is there a rule of thumb for determining the best-proportioned figure?
A. Yes—let your wrist be your guide. I studied a group of models, career professionals, housewives, airline stewardesses, and actresses. Those with well-proportioned figures had one thing in common—their wrist measurement in relation to other parts of their body.

A good example is Pat, a medium-frame model from Alexandria, Virginia, who weighs 125 pounds and is 5 feet 7 inches tall. I measured Pat's wrist. It was 6 inches. For the best-proportioned figure, Pat's ankle should measure one-and-a-half times her wrist, and it did measure 9 inches. Her calf should measure twice her wrist and her thigh three times her wrist. Pat's calf measured 12 inches and her thigh measured 18 inches. Her waist should be four times her wrist, and her hips and bust six times her wrist measurement. Pat's waist was 24 inches, her hips and bust 36 inches.

If your measurements fall within a 3-inch range in certain spots, your body is still well proportioned. For instance, given Pat's 6 inch wrist, the range of measurements for the perfectly proportioned figure would be:

Determining the Well-Proportioned Figure

wrist measurement	6 inches
ankle measurement	8–10 inches
calf measurement	11–13 inches
mid-thigh measurement	17–19 inches
waist measurement	23–26 inches
hip measurement	35–38 inches
bust measurement	34–37 inches

If you are out of proportion, go on my Easy, No-Risk Diet found in the next chapter and exercise regularly, focusing on those areas of your body that are especially troubling you.

If scales scare you, there is a way to determine if you are overweight without getting on them. Professor B. Everard Blanchard of De Paul University in Chicago has developed the following formula:

If you subtract your waist measurement from your height in inches, without shoes, and the result is 36 or greater, you are not too heavy. For instance, in Pat's case you convert her height of 5 feet 7 inches to 67 inches. Subtracting 24 inches for her waistline, you are left with 43 inches. Since 43 is higher than 36, Pat is not overweight. The formula for subtracting waistline from total height will not work, however, for pregnant women or professional athletes who carry a lot of extra muscle.

Now that you know what your goal weight is, you are ready to achieve it.

3

THE

EASY, NO-RISK

DIET

What you'll love about this diet is its variety. Imagine being able to eat pretzels, ice cream, or chocolate chip cookies and not feel you're cheating!

This is an *exchange* diet. That means I have prepared lists of the foods you may eat. Any food on the list has the same caloric content as any other food on the list. *The choice is yours.*

In other words I've taken away the trouble and boredom of counting calories. You don't have to reckon up your calories because I've already done that for you. Just stick to my lists of foods. There is a whole page of goodies, for instance, that can be exchanged for a single piece of bread. Each food on that list has approximately the same number of calories and the same grams of carbohydrates as one slice of bread.

The cardinal aspect of this diet is its flexibility. So many foods are allowed on it that you can individualize. Make it your own. Custom tailor it. Adapt it to your particular life-style. Eat as many times a day as you like.

And while you are enjoying its variety, you will also experience the comfort of knowing you are on a diet that is *nutritious, healthy, and free of the risks to your body that all fad diets harbor.*

Before you go on any diet, including this one, you should get your doctor's permission.

Your health is your most important asset. And your peace of mind is your most important strength. On this diet, you'll be happy knowing that you're doing what's best for your looks and your health at the same time. My diet is specially geared for you to lose at a steady and healthy pace. This will also allow your skin to accommodate the weight loss with the least possible wrinkling. And you will readjust your eating pattern, permanently, developing sound rather than scatter-shot eating habits. It will take about three days to adjust to the diet. At the beginning you may feel like a martyr eating at this new level. But adjust you will, because the diet is easy to follow, and you will experience the profound satisfaction of seeing yourself getting slimmer.

This is an Easy, No-Risk 1,200-calorie diet that really works. It was tried by a group called WON, headed by Dr. Maria Simonson of the School of Public Health at Johns Hopkins Hospital, by some members of the Congressional Wives Club in Washington, D.C., and also by my private patients. The overwhelming majority had the same happy response—*it works and it's easy to stick to.*

Former Maryland Congressman Carlton Sickles, who got the diet from his wife, Simi, a member of the Congressional Wives Club, said it's the easiest diet he has ever been on. Its variety allows him to adjust it to his busy schedule, which includes a lot of eating in restaurants.

The only people who did not lose effectively were patients who had difficulty in burning carbohydrates—people I call

58

carboholics. For them I modified my original diet, decreasing the amount of carbohydrates and increasing the amount of protein, *but keeping the diet nutritionally sound.* If you go on my diet for one week and you *don't* lose weight, you may be a carboholic. *You should consult your doctor* and then with his consent go on my Easy, No-Risk Diet for Carboholics found in Chapter 4.

Ideally, people who need to lose weight should lose an average of one to two pounds a week. The majority of people who tried the diet lost at this rate. Some lost as much as ten pounds in a single week, but much of that was the excess fluid. Your body will quickly adjust to a smaller amount of food and your weight loss will level off. Body weight may fluctuate daily due to water balance. True weight loss is evident when you weigh yourself once a week at the same time before dressing. Studies have shown that dieters who lose more than two pounds a week have trouble keeping them off. *Keeping the weight off is what you want.*

My diet allows you to plan meals according to your life-style. *Three to six meals a day is what I strongly recommend. Don't skip breakfast*—it doesn't work. Skipping breakfast causes hunger for a whole variety of foods later in the day. Whether you eat three, four, five or six meals a day is really up to you. My diet provides you with 70 grams of protein, 47 grams of fat, 129 grams of carbohydrate, and is adequate in vitamins and minerals. Unless you have an illness for which your doctor has prescribed a vitamin, you definitely don't need to take a vitamin pill or minerals on this diet.

It is important that you drink a glass of water before beginning each meal. If you don't like water, then drink another fluid low in calories, such as a glass of iced tea with or without lemon, or a glass of sparkling soda water with or without lemon or lime. If you prefer to drink a hot cup of tea or broth before each meal, that, too, is perfectly acceptable. A cup of broth will satisfy hunger pangs in between meals, too. The idea is simply to get fluid into your stomach so that you will be satisfied eating less. Eating is one of the great pleasures of life and this diet will allow you to enjoy eating in a sensible way.

GENERAL INSTRUCTIONS FOR MY EASY, NO-RISK DIET

● Use only those foods listed. Do not add flour or cornmeal (or Shake and Bake), do not add butter, oil, or cream unless used as a "fat share."

● Meats should be baked, broiled, or roasted. Pam may be used to oil the pan for frying. If food is fried, one fat share must be used, and one bread share may be used if crumbs are desired. Fish should be poached, broiled, or baked. Vegetables should be cooked in salted water. Chicken should be broiled, stewed or baked; turkey roasted. Either chicken or beef bouillon cubes may be added for flavor. Food may be seasoned with some of the fat allowed in the diet and with herbs and spices.

● Vegetables are low in calories and can be used to satisfy those inevitable hunger pangs. Keep a container of cleaned and washed celery sticks, cauliflower rosettes, carrot sticks, broccoli flowers, radishes, cucumbers, cabbage, turnips, mushrooms raw or cooked (boiled or broiled), green pepper rings, or tomatoes in season, for nibbling. Vary the assortment.

● Plan meals ahead and incorporate your meals with those of your family wherever possible.

● Always plan ahead for parties, eat less for lunch and breakfast if you wish, but *do not skip a meal.*

● Always eat sitting at a table. Eat slowly and chew your food well. If you are inclined to eat fast, slow down. Remember, your stomach is twenty minutes ahead of your brain. In other words, from the time you put food into your mouth and it arrives in your stomach until your brain responds by saying, "I've had enough," there is a twenty-minute time lag. So each meal should last at least twenty minutes.

• Fruit used should either be fresh or canned without sugar. Water-packed fruit is available in all supermarkets.

• Diet sodas may be used. You may drink up to twenty-four ounces of diet sodas a day. If you are caffeine sensitive, see page 176 for the amount of caffeine in various cola drinks. Read labels to be sure there is no sugar. At a party ask for a diet soda with a twist of lemon.

• It is important to eat at least three meals daily, spaced about four to five hours apart. Some people find it easier to reduce their calorie intake by having six small meals. Others find three meals with a snack results in better weight loss and less hunger. Experiment to determine which route suits you best. Never exceed the daily 1,200-calorie food intake. Do not omit foods. All are needed for good nutrition.

• Don't forget exercise. Walk whenever you can instead of driving. Park farther away from your destination and walk. Follow the TV guide for exercise shows, take out a membership in your local Y or gym, learn to play tennis, or swim. Find some form of exercise you enjoy. Daily moderate exercise will do more for you than a single all-out and exhausting once-a-week effort. Try to choose some pleasurable way to exercise—yoga, a dance class, or tennis with in-between practice, or just a daily walk or bike ride can be renewing and burn up calories as well.

It is important for you to realize that the amounts of food allowed in each group in my Easy, No-Risk Diet are listed as "amount per average serving" and not as calories. You need not count your calories since I have already done this for you. All you have to do is limit yourself to the amount indicated and allowed. Any food which is not mentioned on my Easy, No-Risk Diet is not allowed unless approved by your doctor.

EASY, NO-RISK DIET

Daily food intake for my 1,200-calorie diet: See lists for amounts of food.

SIX PROTEIN SHARES

THREE FRUIT SHARES

TWO DAIRY SHARES

THREE FAT SHARES

FIVE BREAD SHARES

VEGETABLES THAT ARE LISTED MAY BE USED AS DESIRED

Protein Shares

Eat Six Easy, No-Risk Protein Shares Each Day

	Measure
Meat and poultry (moderate fat) (beef, veal, lamb, pork, liver, etc.)	1 ounce
Cold cuts (4½ inches square, ⅛ inch thick)	1 slice
Frankfurters (8–9 to the pound)	1
Fish, any kind	1 oz.
Salmon, tuna, crab, lobster	¼ cup
Oysters, shrimp, clams	5 small
Sardines (well drained)	3 medium
Cheese,	1 ounce
Cottage cheese, creamed	¼ cup
Egg	1
Peanut butter*	2 tablespoons

Example—you could use any of the following portions to fulfill your 6 protein shares:

One 6-ounce steak
or 3 ounces lamb, 1 frankfurter and 2
ounces (½ cup) cottage cheese
or 1 egg, ¼ cup tuna, and 4 ounces ground beef

The combinations are up to you. Just be sure you don't go over the amount allowed—your total protein eaten in one day must be exactly 6 protein shares.

*Limit use to 2 tablespoons a day

Fruit Shares

Eat Three Easy No-Risk Fruit Shares Each Day Without Added Sugar—Or Canned, Water-Packed Fruits

Apple	1 small (2 inch diam.)
Apple juice	⅓ cup
Applesauce	½ cup
Apricots (dried)	4 halves
Apricots (fresh or water-packed)	2 medium
Banana	½ small
*Berries (black, raspberries and strawberries)	1 cup
Blueberries (fresh or water-packed)	cup
*Cantaloupe	¼ (6-inch diam.)
Cherries (Bing)	10 large
Cherries (Royal Anne)	12
Dates	2
Figs (fresh or water-packed)	2 large
Figs (dried)	1 small
Fruit cocktail (water-packed)	½ cup
*Grapefruit	½ small
*Grapefruit juice	½ cup
*Grapefruit sections	½ cup
Grapes	12 large
Grapes (seedless)	24 small

Grape juice	¼ cup
Guava	¼ medium
Honeydew melon	⅛ (7-inch diam.)
*Mango	½ small
Nectarine	1 medium
*Orange	1 small
*Orange juice	½ cup
*Orange (mandarin, water-packed)	1½ cups
*Papaya	⅓ medium
Peach (fresh or water-packed)	1 medium
Pear (fresh or water-packed)	1 small
Pineapple (fresh or water-packed)	½ cup
Pineapple (water-packed)	2 slices
Pineapple juice	⅓ cup
Plantain	1½-inch long slice
Plums (fresh or water-packed)	2 medium
Prune juice	¼ cup
Prunes (dried)	2 medium
Raisins	2 tablespoons
*Tangerine	1 large
*Tomato juice or V-8 juice	1 cup
Watermelon (without rind)	1 cup
Watermelon (with rind)	½ round, 1 inch thick

*These fruits are excellent sources of vitamin C and one source should be included every day.

Dairy Shares

Have Two Easy, No-Risk Dairy Shares Each Day

	Measure
Milk, evaporated, skim	½ cup
Milk, powdered skim, reconstituted	1 cup
Buttermilk	1 cup
Milk, skim	1 cup
Yogurt made with skim milk	1 cup

A pint (or two cups) of skim milk is recommended daily to supply adequate protein, carbohydrate, vitamins, and calcium. Those of you who do not care for skim milk may substitute 1 cup of whole milk for 1 cup of skim milk. However, if you do this, you must give up 1 fat share.

1 cup whole milk = 1 cup skim milk plus 1 fat share.

If you drink coffee, try heating part of your skim milk and pour in as you pour the coffee into your cup for a satisfying café au lait.

If you do not like milk at all, you may substitute the following low-fat cheese for 1 cup skim milk.

    1 ounce Edam
    1 ounce Liederkranz
    1 ounce mysost
    1 ounce sapsago
    1 ounce Neufchatel
    1 ounce mozzarella
    6 tablespoons cottage cheese, uncreamed

On my Easy, No-Risk Diet and my Easy, No-Risk Diet for Carboholics (Chapter 4) you may substitute the following cheeses for one cup of skim milk. You must also give up ½ fat share. In other words, 1 cup skim milk plus ½ fat share equals:

1 ounce Cheddar
1 ounce domestic blue cheese or Stilton
1 ounce Camembert
3½ ounces or 6 tablespoons cottage cheese, creamed
1 ounce Gruyère
1 ounce Parmesan
1 ounce Roquefort
1 ounce Swiss (domestic or imported)
1 ounce Monterey Jack
1 ounce Fontina
1 ounce Gorgonzola
1 ounce Gouda

On all the Figure-Keeper Plans you do not have to give up ½ fat share when you exchange one cup of skim milk for the cheese list above.

Hints on Skim Milk

It is best to use powdered skim milk because it has the least amount of fat. Follow the directions on the label and refrigerate for at least two hours before using to improve the flavor. Skim milk can also be whipped—again follow the directions on the package. (The secret to whipping is to have the beater and bowl ice-cold.)

If you find mixing milk too time-consuming, purchase regular 1 percent butterfat skimmed milk from your supplier.

Fat Shares
Eat Three Easy, No-Risk Fat Shares Each Day

Avocado (4-inch diam.)	⅛
Butter or margarine	1 teaspoon
Bacon (crisp)	1 slice
Cream, light (18 percent butterfat)	2 tablespoons
Cream, heavy (32 percent butterfat)	1 tablespoon
Cream, sour	2 tablespoons
Cream cheese	1 tablespoon
French dressing	1 tablespoon
Half and Half	3 tablespoons
Mayonnaise	1 teaspoon
Nuts	6 small
Oil or cooking fat	1 teaspoon
Olives (ripe)	5 small (limit to 1 fat share)
Olives (green)	10 medium (limit to 1 fat share)

Bread Shares
Have Five Easy, No-Risk Bread Shares Each Day

You may substitute any of the following for 1 slice of bread:

BREAD AND BREAD PRODUCTS:

Bagel	½
*Biscuits	1
Bread, enriched, whole grain, raisin	1 slice
*Cornbread (2-inch square, 1-inch thick)	1
*Muffin (small)	1
Muffin, English	½
Pancake (4-inch diam.)	1
Roll, dinner small	1
Hamburger or hard roll	½
Hot dog roll	1
*Tortilla	1
Waffle (5-inch diam.)	½

*Omit 1 fat share

CAKES AND COOKIES—UNICED:

Angel food (18-slice cake/10-inch cake)	1 piece
Plain (mix-20 pieces/9-inch cake)	1 piece
*Pound (½-inch slice)	1
*Doughnuts	
Frozen—Morton's sugar & spice	1
Shortbread cookies (1½–2-inch square)	2
Butter Thin cookies (2½-inch square)	2
Pepperidge Farm Pirouettes, vanilla	2
Chocolate chip (1½-inch diam.)	2
Fruitana raisin	1
Small ginger or lemon snaps	5
Plain oatmeal (2-inch diam.)	1
*Pop-ups	½
Sugar (2-inch diam.)	1
Vanilla wafers (small)	6

*Omit 1 fat share

CEREALS AND VEGETABLE STARCHES:

Cereal (cooked)	½ cup
*Cereal (dry: flake or puffed)	¾ cup
Corn (½ large ear)	⅓ cup
Dried beans and peas (cooked)	½ cup
Grits, rice, noodles, spaghetti, all pasta (cooked)	½ cup
Lima beans	½ cup
†Onion rings (frozen)	2 ounces
Parsnips	⅔ cup
Potatoes: Baked white (2-inch diam.)	1 small
**French fries (frozen) (5 pieces, ½-inch diam., 3-inches long)	2 ounces
†Potato puffs	6
Sweet or yam	¼ cup

*Cereals prepared with dried fruit, sugar, coconut, honey, or nuts are not allowed
†Omit 2 fat shares
**Omit 1 fat share

CRACKERS:

Animal	8
Bread sticks (3-inches long), cheese, onion, garlic	6
Cinnamon crisp (smallest score)	4
Cocoa grahams	3
Holland rusk	½
Honey grahams (smallest score)	4
Matzo (6-inch square) plain	⅔
Melba Toast 3 X 2 inches	5
Oyster	25
*Peanut butter or cheese (Sandwich type ⅞ ounce)	1 package
Pretzels: Dutch or soft	1
Small 3 ring	6
Veri thin ¾ ounce	70
Round thin	7
Rye Krisp	3
Saltines	5
Sea Toast	1
Soda	3
Triscuit	4
Zwieback	3

*Omit 1 fat share

ICE CREAM AND DESSERTS:

*Chocolate covered ice cream bar	1
†Chocolate covered ice milk bar	1
Fudge Bar	1
†Ice Cream—chocolate, vanilla, strawberry	½ cup
†Ice milk	½ cup
Ice cream cone (not sugar) empty	1
Twin Popsicle	1
†Ice cream sandwich (reg. size)	½
Ice cream sandwich (mini)	1
Orange cream bar	1
Sherbet	⅓ cup
Toffee crunch bar	1
Water ice	¼ cup
Jello	½ cup

*Omit 2 fat shares
†Omit 1 fat share

*Cheese Tid Bits (Nab)	50
†Fritos	1 ounce
Popcorn, popped (use fat shares for seasoning)	1½ cups
*Potato chips	15 chips

*Omit 1 fat share
†Omit 2 fat shares

VEGETABLES
NO LIMIT. USE FRESH, FROZEN, OR CANNED

Asparagus
Bean sprouts
Beet greens
Beets
Broccoli*
Brussels sprouts*
Cabbage (all kinds)
Carrots
Cauliflower
Celery
Chard
Chicory
Collard greens*
Cucumber
Dandelion greens
Eggplant
Endive
Escarole
Green beans
Kale
Kohlrabi
Leeks

Lettuce
Mushrooms
Mustard greens*
Onions
Okra
Oyster plant
Peas
Peppers
Poke
Pumpkin
Radishes
Rutabagas
Sauerkraut
Spinach*
Squash (winter)
Tomatoes*
Turnip greens*
Turnips
Water chestnuts
Watercress
Wax beans

*These vegetables are excellent sources of vitamin C and one source should be included daily. Have a green leafy or yellow vegetable each day to supply vitamin A.

Foods Allowed as Desired

Coffee
Tea
Clear broth
Bouillon (without fat) low salt
  preferable
Gelatin (unsweetened)
Rennet Tablets
Lemon
Rhubarb
D-Zerta gelatin
Puddings, without sugar,
  made with the skim milk
  allowed on the diet
Mustard
Pickles (sour)
Pickles (unsweetened dill)
Artificial sweetenings
Pepper
Spices
Vinegar
Cranberries (unsweetened)

Alcohol Shares

Give up 2½ fat shares for: 1½-ounce jigger whisky, rye, scotch, bourbon, rum, vodka, gin; or one 8-ounce glass beer or 3½ ounces sweet wine.

Give up 2 fat shares for: 1 8-ounce glass ale, 1 4-ounce glass champagne, or 3½ ounces dry wine, white or red, Sauterne, domestic sherry.

Q. **I'm often desperate during the day for something sweet. Have you any suggestions for satisfying that sweet yen without making havoc of my daily shares allowance?**

A. Yes, this is an especially besetting problem for dieters, and in response to a legion of requests I've developed a Super Shake. You can make it the night before and put it in the refrigerator for the next day's sweet craving. If you're going out, just take the shake along with you in a thermos—it will keep for the entire day.

Super Shake

1 cup skim milk

1 fruit share (any fresh fruit or frozen fruit without sugar; with fresh fruit use 3 ice cubes; these are not required with frozen fruit)

2 tablespoons skim milk cottage cheese (optional)

2 drops artificial sweetener (if additional sweetness is desired)

Make shake in blender and keep in the refrigerator. This exchanges for 1 dairy share, 1 fruit share, and 1 protein share on your daily allowance.

Below are two Easy, No-Risk Diet Meal Plans, including one for eggwatchers:

PATTERN MEAL

Plan A: For Non-Eggwatchers
(See pages 64 through 73 for size of servings of food.)

A. 1 serving fruit

M. *1 egg, any style—not fried unless allowed in diet
1 teaspoon butter or substitute a fat share
1 slice bread or 1 bread share
Coffee or tea if desired

N 2 ounces meat or 2 protein shares
O Vegetables
O 1 fat share
N 1 serving fruit
2 bread shares
1 cup skim milk or buttermilk
Coffee or tea if desired

3 ounces meat or 3 protein shares
Vegetables
P. 1 fat share
M. 1 serving fruit
1 bread share
Coffee or tea if desired

S 1 bread share
N 1 cup skim milk
A
C
K

*Prudent men should limit eggs to no more than four per week. Women, until they no longer have monthly menstrual periods, can have four to seven eggs per week to supply needed iron. There are several tasty egg substitutes available for cholesterol watchers: Egg Beater's, Cono, Eggstra, and Ova-Comp. Read labels for directions and substitute for the egg listed.

Plan B: For Eggwatchers
(See pages 64 through 73 for size of servings of food.)

A.	1 serving fruit
M.	1 serving cereal
	1 teaspoon butter or substitute
	1 slice bread or 1 bread share
	1 cup skim milk or buttermilk
	Coffee or tea if desired

N	2 ounces meat or 2 protein shares
O	Vegetables
O	1 serving fruit
N	2 bread shares
	½ cup skim milk or buttermilk
	Coffee or tea if desired

P.	4 ounces meat or 4 protein shares
M.	Vegetables
	1 fat share
	1 serving fruit
	Coffee or tea if desired

S	1 bread share
N	½ cup skim milk or buttermilk or dairy share
A	
C	
K	

If the menu for a meal contains a food you don't like, consult the exchange lists (pages 64 through 73) and select one that appeals to you. You can interchange fruits, or make substitutions for the bread, or substitutions for milk from the dairy list. If the meat does not suit you, select something else from the protein shares list. Look at the fat shares list for substitutions. *The beauty of this diet is that you can select foods that are your favorites—forget about counting calories. This is done for you.*

SUGGESTED WEEK OF EASY, NO-RISK MENUS

Sunday

B R E A K F A S T

½ cup orange juice
1 egg poached on toast with 1 teaspoon butter or
    margarine
Coffee or tea if desired

L U N C H

10 small shrimp on lettuce with tomato wedges,
    celery, dill pickle chips, diet dressing
1 English muffin
1 teaspoon butter or margarine
½ apple
1 cup skim milk or buttermilk
Coffee or tea if desired

D I N N E R

3 ounces tenderloin steak, broiled
Asparagus spears
Cauliflower with lemon and paprika
Tossed green salad with diet dressing
1 teaspoon butter
1 small dinner roll
Fresh pear
Coffee or tea if desired

S N A C K

4 graham crackers
1 cup skim milk

Monday

B		⅓ cup pineapple juice
R	**F**	¾ cup puffed wheat
E	**A**	½ cup skim milk
A	**S**	1 slice toast
K	**T**	1 teaspoon butter
		Coffee or tea if desired

L
U
N
C
H

Beef bouillon
½ cup cottage cheese on lettuce with 1 fresh peach or
   2 halves of canned peaches, water-packed
½ English muffin, toasted
1 teaspoon butter or margarine
Coffee or tea if desired

M S
I N
D A
D C
A K
Y

6 vanilla wafers
½ cup skim milk
Few drops almond flavoring
Artificial sweetener if desired   } Whip in blender
1–2 ice cubes

D
I
N
N
E
R

*½ pan broiled chicken breast with herbs
Broiled tomato
Fresh green beans with water chestnuts
1 teaspoon margarine or butter (season vegetables)
Lettuce heart with lo-cal dressing
D-Zerta gelatin with ½ banana
Coffee or tea if desired

B T S
E I N
D M A
** E C**
**   K**

1 slice American cheese
4 Triscuits
1 cup skim milk

*Pan broiled chicken: Rub chicken with soy sauce. Place in pan on low heat (electric frying pan at 230°). Brown with skin side down, turning until evenly brown. Cover and cook until tender (about 30–35 minutes).

Tuesday

B R E A K F A S T

½ grapefruit
1 egg coddled with 1 tablespoon milk salt, pepper
¼ teaspoon butter
1 slice whole wheat toast
¾ teaspoon butter
Coffee or tea if desired

L U N C H

Tuna salad with ½ cup tuna fish—water-packed, chopped celery, chopped green pepper, peas. Toss with 1 tablespoon mayonnaise—serve on lettuce
1 English muffin, toasted
½ cup pineapple, fresh, water-packed, 2 slices
1 cup milk, skim

D I N N E R

1 double lamb chop, broiled
Baked potato with 2 tablespoons sour cream or 1 teaspoon butter
Peas with mushrooms
Sliced orange salad with fresh mint garnish
D-Zerta pudding made with ½ cup skim milk
Coffee or tea if desired

S N A C K

¾ cup cornflakes
½ cup skim milk

Wednesday

BREAKFAST

½ cup orange juice
½ cup oatmeal
1 slice toast
1 teaspoon butter or margarine
½ cup skim milk
Coffee or tea if desired

LUNCH

1 cup jellied consomme, lemon wedge
1 slice Swiss cheese ⅛-inch thick
1 slice baked ham ⅛-inch thick
Sauerkraut
Kosher dill pickles
1 slice rye bread—toast bread and
run sandwich under broiler
Small apple
½ cup skim milk
Iced tea

DINNER

4-ounce salmon steak with lemon and rosemary
Broccoli
Boiled new potatoes, 1 small, 2-inch diameter
Roll
Coleslaw with diet dressing
2 teaspoons butter or margarine
1 tangerine
Coffee or tea if desired

SNACK

3 cocoa grahams
1 cup skim milk

Thursday

B		1 shredded wheat biscuit
R	**F**	½ sliced banana
E	**A**	1 slice toast
A	**S**	1 teaspoon butter or margarine
K	**T**	Coffee or tea if desired
		1 cup skim milk

L	Sandwich with 2 slices bologna—each ⅛-inch thick
U	2 slices rye bread with lettuce and mustard
N	2 teaspoons mayonnaise
C	Celery sticks
H	Carrot sticks
	Dill pickle
	Diet soda

D	4 ounces lean chopped sirloin, broiled
I	Spinach with ½ to 1 teaspoon vinegar
N	Stewed tomatoes with ⅓ cup kernel corn
N	Perfection salad in lime D-Zerta
E	(chopped cabbage, green pepper, pimento)
R	Coffee or tea if desired
	½ broiled grapefruit, flavored with 1 teaspoon sherry

S	1 cup skim milk
N	1 cup strawberries
A	Artificial sweetener and 2 ice cubes—blend for
C	"shake"
K	

Friday

B **R** **E** **A** **K** **F** **A** **S** **T**	½ grapefruit ¾ cup Wheaties ½ cup skim milk 1 slice toast 1 teaspoon butter or margarine Coffee or tea if desired
L **U** **N** **C** **H**	½ cup crab meat on lettuce—lemon wedge 1 teaspoon mayonnaise cucumber sticks 5 pieces Melba toast Coffee or tea ½ cup D-Zerta pudding, made with skim milk
D **I** **N** **N** **E** **R**	Chicken broth 4 ounces baked veal chop with onion rings, mushrooms* Small baked potato 1 teaspoon butter or margarine Green and wax beans Tossed salad with lo-cal dressing ½ banana in strawberry D-Zerta Coffee or tea if desired
S **N** **A** **C** **K**	6 gingersnaps 1½ inches diameter 1 cup skim milk

*Brown chops over low heat, using Pam. Season, add sliced tomatoes, onion, and mushrooms. Cover and bake in oven 350° for 45 minutes or until tender.

Saturday

BREAKFAST

1 cup tomato juice
1 egg on one slice toast
1 slice crisp bacon
Coffee or tea if desired

LUNCH

½ cup cottage cheese on lettuce with 4 halves
    water-packed apricots
3 Rye Krisp
1 cup skim milk or buttermilk

DINNER

3 ounces beef cubes (see page 85) braised on ½ cup
    cooked noodles
Spinach
Sliced tomato salad on endive, use any low-calorie
dressing or one we give on page 109.
1 fat share
1 small dinner roll
Fresh pear
Coffee or tea if desired

SNACK

6 small 3-ring pretzels
1 cup skim milk

PATTERN MEAL PLAN FOR 6 MEALS DAILY

If you prefer eating six small meals a day, this sample six meal, 1,200-calorie pattern is for you:

B R E A K F A S T
Fruit or juice—or 1 fruit share
Cereal—1 bread share
½ cup skim milk
Coffee or tea if desired

M I D M O R N I N G
1 slice toast
1 teaspoon butter or margarine
Tea or coffee if desired

L U N C H
½ sandwich (using 2 slices bread, 2 ounces meat or cheese and 1 teaspoon fat share)
Salad with low-calorie dressing
8 ounces skim milk (see dairy list)

M I D D D A Y S N A C K
½ sandwich (from lunch)
1 fruit share
Tea or coffee if desired

D I N N E R
4 protein shares
Vegetables
Bouillon
Salad—low-calorie dressing
1 fat share

B E D T I M E S N A C K
4 ounces skim milk—see dairy list
1 bread share
1 fruit share

COOKING HINTS FOR LOSING WEIGHT

Several cookbooks for dieters are available that offer useful hints and recipes for preparing interesting foods, low in calories. Among them are *Better Homes and Gardens' Eat and Stay Slim*, published by the Meredith Press, New York, and the *Ladies' Home Journal*'s *Family Diet Book* by Evan Frances, published by the Macmillan Publishing Co., New York. Your local library will have others.

How to Prepare Meats, Fish, and Poultry

Ground meat patties, cubes of beef, veal, lamb, or pork can be browned in a heavy frying pan without additional fat. Begin at a low temperature and the meat will brown and cook in its own juices, or if it is too dry, add 2 tablespoons of water or broth. Add salt, pepper, and your favorite spices or herbs after the meat is browned. Try Pam if sticking is a problem or use a Teflon-lined pan.

Braising can be done by browning beef, lamb, or pork cubes as noted above, then adding herbs, tomato puree, or canned tomatoes prepared in a blender (for one serving use ½ to ¾ cup), chopped onions, chopped green peppers, and a bit of water if necessary. Cover tightly and cook on top of the stove until done, or in the oven at 350°F. Usually an hour's cooking is sufficient. Don't forget spices or herbs (sweet basil, rosemary, marjoram, thyme, and oregano—to name a few). You'll want to check occasionally to be sure there is sufficient liquid. Add water or bouillon as necessary.

Barbecuing over charcoal is another way to cook meat patties, shish kebab, chicken, etc. Once again you'll want to make sure your fire is not too hot.

Make a barbecue sauce either in your blender, or if you have no blender, mix with a hand beater in a bowl. (This will take care of 1½ pounds of meat or poultry and is easily doubled.)

Barbecue Sauce

1 cup tomato puree or canned tomatoes
½ cup vinegar or lemon juice
1 teaspoon salt
½ teaspoon paprika
¼ teaspoon ginger or curry powder
½ teaspoon basil or oregano
Artificial sweetener to taste

Marinate beef cubes, chicken, lamb cubes, or pork cubes for at least 4 hours or overnight in the refrigerator. Place cubes on skewer for broiling, or chicken on rack. Baste with remaining sauce during cooking.

Fish may be pan fried in part of the daily fat shares allowance, or the pan may be sprayed with Pam. Fish filets, for example, sole or flounder, may be broiled by spreading the fish with mayonnaise (as part of your fat shares allowance) sprinkled with paprika, and broiled under the oven broiler until brown—10 to 15 minutes. The filets may be garnished with sliced olives to add eye appeal. Squeezing lemon juice on your fish perks up its flavor.

If you're not crazy about cottage cheese, you might learn to like it by improving the taste. Try adding one of these, and mix in thoroughly:

—snipped chives (fresh or frozen)
—dill
—caraway seeds
—parsley
—curry powder
—chopped green pepper
—chopped radishes
—chopped carrots

You will taste a delicious difference.

How to Prepare Vegetables

Vegetables should be cooked without adding additional calories. However, some of the daily fat shares allowance on the diet may be used to season. Green vegetables cooked in beef bouillon are refreshing (consult cookbook for timing instructions). Try broccoli, Brussels sprouts, spinach, collard greens, and kale this way.

Combinations of vegetables are also pleasing. Have you tried carrots and onions together? Green beans or peas with mushrooms? Green beans with tomatoes and cauliflower are also interesting. Don't forget herbs and spices (your cookbook will give you suggestions). They are calorie-free. Don't overseason, though—just enough to enhance the flavor of the vegetable is the best guide. You'll find vegetable cookery a great adventure.

Be an original cook. Try some of these vegetable seasoning hints. A little seasoning goes a long way—add just a sprinkle to the entire recipe, taste, and add more to suit your taste.

Asparagus: caraway seed, mustard, sesame seed, tarragon
Green beans: basil, bay leaves, curry, dill, marjoram, mustard, oregano, savory, sesame seed, tarragon, thyme
Lima beans: celery seed, chili powder, curry, oregano, sage
Broccoli: caraway seed, mustard, oregano
Brussels sprouts: caraway seed, mustard, nutmeg, sage
Cabbage: allspice, basil, caraway seed, celery seed, dill, mustard, nutmeg, oregano, savory, tarragon

Carrots: allspice, bay leaves, caraway seed, celery seed, chives, curry, dill, ginger, mace, marjoram, mint, nutmeg, savory, tarragon, thyme

Cauliflower: caraway seed, celery seed, curry, dill, mustard, nutmeg, oregano, savory, tarragon

Corn: celery seed, chili powder, chives

Eggplant: allspice, basil, bay leaves, chili powder, marjoram, sage, thyme

Mushrooms: rosemary, tarragon, thyme

Onions: basil, bay leaves, caraway seed, chili powder, curry, ginger, mustard, nutmeg, oregano, sage, thyme

Peas: basil, chili powder, dill, marjoram, mint, mustard, oregano, rosemary, sage

Potatoes, sweet: allspice, cardamom, cinnamon, cloves, ginger, nutmeg

Potatoes, white: basil, bay leaves, caraway seed, celery seed, chives, dill, mace, mustard, oregano, rosemary, savory, sesame seed, thyme

Spinach: allspice, basil, cinnamon, dill, mace, marjoram, nutmeg, oregano, rosemary, sesame seed

Squash, summer: basil, bay leaves, mace, marjoram, mustard, rosemary

Squash, winter: allspice, basil, cinnamon, cloves, ginger, nutmeg

Tomatoes: basil, bay leaves, caraway seed, celery seed, curry, dill, oregano, rosemary, sage, sesame seed, thyme

Turnips: allspice, caraway seed, celery seed, dill, oregano

HINTS FOR THOSE WHO MUST CUT DOWN ON CHOLESTEROL AND SATURATED FAT

We know that overweight people, those who smoke, and those whose families have heart disease are more likely to have heart trouble. The National Institute of Health recommends that individuals prone to heart disease (your physician can advise you) change the type and amount of fat used in their daily diet. Of particular concern are saturated fats and cholesterol. Although the Easy, No-Risk Diet is already low in fat, you may wish to change the type of fat used to mainly polyunsaturated fat.

Some guidelines to control your intake of cholesterol and saturated fat:

• Limit egg yolks to 3 per week, including those used in cooking. Egg substitutes may be used according to instructions on the package.

• Shrimp, high-fat cheese and organ meats such as sweetbreads, liver, and brains are very high in cholesterol. To satisfy an occasional craving, 2 ounces of these may be substituted for 1 egg yolk.

• Use fish, chicken, turkey, and veal as often as possible. Limit beef, lamb, and pork to moderate-size portions, once a day. Lean, well-trimmed meats should be used. Use choice grade or lower; prime costs more and has more fat.

• Meats, poultry, and fish may be baked, broiled, roasted, stewed, or boiled. All meat drippings should be discarded. Meat or poultry skins should not be eaten.

• Restrict use of luncheon rolls or loaves and "variety meats" (sausage, hot dogs) to occasional treats.

• Use vegetable oils and soft margarines that are rich in polyunsaturated fats in place of butter and other cooking fats that are solid or hydrogenated. Read the labels.

- Use skimmed milk and skimmed milk cheese *in place* of those made with whole milk. (See list pages 67 and 68.) Use special fat-controlled high-protein, low-cholesterol cheese or Cheddar cheese substituted for 1 egg yolk. Creamed cottage cheese may also be used *in place* of a serving of meat.
- Nuts may be used with the exception of cashew and macadamia or coconut. (Peanut butter may be used.)
- Use plain breads and rolls *in place* of biscuits, muffins, pancakes, waffles.
- Select desserts from the following: fruits, jello, skim milk puddings, sherbets, water ice, or angel food cake.
- Last but not least, you may have one glass of wine, beer, or a drink mixed with water or soda as often as three times a week. To do this you must give up some fat exchange for that day. (See page 73 for alcohol shares). Did you know that alcohol is metabolized like fat? This means that by weight there are over twice as many calories in alcohol as there are in carbohydrates.

THE FIGURE-KEEPER PLAN: ONCE YOU HAVE LOST WEIGHT HOW TO KEEP IT OFF

This section should be read when you have achieved your ideal weight.

Maintaining your weight loss is the true test of a successful weight-reducing adventure. During the weight-loss period new eating habits should have become a new way of life for you. Let's face it—you will never be able to eat as freely as your naturally slender friend. Keep a diary of your eating patterns, including weekly weight and a daily notation of what, when, where, and with whom you eat, as well as your state of mind. Weigh yourself once a week, and remember that any gain should prompt you to return to the diet until your new weight gain is lost.

FIGURE-KEEPER PLAN*

EIGHT PROTEIN SHARES

THREE FRUIT SHARES

TWO DAIRY SHARES

FIVE FAT SHARES

SIX BREAD SHARES

VEGETABLES THAT ARE LISTED MAY BE USED AS DESIRED

*(See shares lists pages 64 through 73.)

Your Figure-Keeper Diet allows you to eat more than you did on the basic 1,200-calorie diet to *lose* weight. Yet, as you will see, both are flexible diets which allow you freedom to make choices and keep eating interestingly.

Following are two suggested meal plans to get you thinking in a slightly bigger meal pattern. Note: This diet has approximately 1,800 calories, 100 grams protein, 75 grams fat, 180 grams carbohydrates.

PATTERN MEAL PLAN
Plan A

B		1 serving fruit
R	**F**	1 egg—any style
E	**A**	1 bread share
A	**S**	1 teaspoon butter or margarine
K	**T**	1 cup of skim milk
		Coffee or tea if desired
		1 tablespoon cream and 1 teaspoon sugar if desired

L	Two protein shares
U	1 serving vegetable
N	Salad if desired
C	2 teaspoon butter or margarine (2 fat shares)
H	2 bread shares
	1 serving of fruit or dessert
	Coffee or tea if desired
	1 tablespoon cream and 1 teaspoon of sugar if desired

D	Four protein shares
I	2 servings vegetables
N	Salad if desired
N	2 fat shares
E	2 bread shares
R	1 serving of fruit or dessert
	Coffee or tea if desired
	1 tablespoon cream and 1 teaspoon sugar if desired

S	1 protein share
N	1 bread share
A	1 cup skim milk
C	
K	

Q. I prefer not to eat so many eggs. Can you design a Figure-Keeper Plan that takes this into consideration?

A. Plan B does exactly that. Remember, for proper servings of food see exchange list.

PATTERN MEAL PLAN
Plan B: For Eggwatchers

B		1 serving fruit
R	**F**	1 serving cereal
E	**A**	1 bread share
A	**S**	1 teaspoon butter or margarine
K	**T**	1 cup skim milk
		Coffee or tea if desired
		1 tablespoon cream and 1 teaspoon sugar if desired

L	3 protein shares
U	1 serving of vegetable
N	Salad if desired
C	2 teaspoon butter or margarine (2 fat shares)
H	2 bread shares
	1 serving of fruit or dessert
	Coffee or tea if desired
	1 tablespoon cream and 1 teaspoon sugar if desired

D	4 protein shares
I	Two servings of vegetable
N	Salad if desired
N	2 fat shares
E	1 serving of fruit or dessert
R	Coffee or tea if desired
	1 tablespoon cream and 1 teaspoon sugar if desired

S	1 protein share
N	1 bread share
A	1 cup skim milk
C	
K	

If cholesterol is a problem for you, see instruction for control on pages 89 and 90.

GENERAL DIRECTIONS FOR FIGURE-KEEPER
PLAN DIET

Meat may be broiled, roasted, stewed, braised, or occasionally fried. Vegetables should be cooked in clear salted water, or simply prepared in combination with each other—consult your favorite cookbook for interesting and new ideas. Seldom fry—½ cup is a serving.

Fruit may be fresh, dried, or canned. Follow your fruit list, but canned fruits may be used that have been canned with sugar (light syrup only). Read the labels.

Desserts may occasionally be added to the diet—not more than one a day. Servings are as follows:

⅛ of 9-inch pie
½ cup of any pudding
1/12 of 10-inch cake or 2-inch square
3 cookies 2 inches in diameter

Q. I went on your Figure-Keeper Plan and gained weight. What should I do?

A. You should reduce your intake of desserts, use fruit without sugar, and eliminate sugar and cream from the diet plan. If you can't shed the additional weight, return to the strict 1,200-calorie diet.

Q. May I have an occasional alcoholic beverage?

A. You may substitute for alcoholic beverages according to basic shares list pages 64 through 73. Remember that these are "empty calories."

Q. Can I have cream and sugar with my coffee?

A. The meal plans mention limited use of cream and sugar in coffee or tea. If you have missed having cream and sugar in your beverages you can try having it again, but do not exceed the amount of 1 tablespoon of cream or half & half (saves calories). If your artificial sweetener is satisfying to you, continue using it.

Q. I got used to and like my low-calorie salad dressing. Can I continue to use it?

A. Also mentioned in the meal plan is low-calorie dressing for salads. Once again, if you are satisfied with your selection, it certainly saves calories and will help you maintain your weight loss.

Q. I like the convenience of canned soups. How can I exchange them?

A. It can be done easily.

CONDENSED SOUPS IN SHARES LISTS

The following share food lists have been prepared by the Campbell Soup Company, based on the Standard Exchange Units set forth by the American Dietetic Association, the American Diabetic Association, and the Public Health Service, Department of Health, Education and Welfare.

We in no way endorse any specific brand name products. They are listed because Campbell is the only soup company we know that publishes a list, and because many people use soups.

Recommendations for Placing Campbell's Soups* into Shares Lists

---

Exchange for
1 bread and ½ fat share

Asparagus, Cream of
Tomato

Exchange for
1½ bread share and ½ protein share

Beef Noodle
Curley Noodle with Chicken
Turkey Noodle

Exchange for
1 bread and ½ protein shares

Tomato Beef Noodle

Exchange for
¼ protein and ½ bread shares

Chicken Gumbo
Chicken Noodle
Chicken Noodle-O's
Chicken with Rice
Chicken with Stars

Exchange for
½ bread and 1 fat shares

Celery, Cream of
Chicken, Cream of
Mushroom, Golden

Exchange for
1 protein and 1½ bread shares

Split Pea with Ham

---

*These recommendations are based on a 1 cup portion.

Other products that you may serve but do not need to measure are:
Beef Broth
Consommé
Tomato Juice
"V-8" Cocktail Vegetable Juice

96

For the Figure-Keeper Diet, the Campbell Ready to Serve Soups and canned products, Franco-American canned products, and Swanson Brand Frozen prepared products may be used. Shares must be used as noted. For those requiring a substitution for "B Vegetables" see the list.

B Vegetables include:

Beets	Peas (green)
Carrots	Pumpkin
Kohlrabi	Rutabagas
Onions	Squash (winter)
Oyster Plant	Turnips

These vegetables should not be used in combination with those products listing a substitution for B vegetables.

Any other vegetables may be used.

Campbell's Canned Products*

**Exchange Substitution for
1½ bread, 1 vegetable B, and ½ fat shares**

Home Style Beans

**Exchange Substitution for
1½ bread and ½ protein shares**

Pork & Beans with Tomato Sauce

**Exchange Substitution for
1¼ bread, 1 vegetable B, and ½ fat shares**

Beans & Franks in Tomato
& Molasses Sauce

**Exchange Substitution for
1¼ bread, 1 vegetable B, and ½ fat shares**

Barbecue Beans
Old Fashioned Beans in Molasses
and Brown Sugar Sauce

**Exchange Substitution for
1 bread and 1 protein shares**

Beans 'n Beef in Tomato Sauce

*1 Cup Portion

Exchange Substitution for
1½ bread, 1½ protein, and 1 vegetable
B shares

Chunky Split Pea with Ham

Exchange Substitution for
1 bread, 1 protein, ½ fat, and ½
vegetable B shares

Chunky Sirloin Burger

Exchange Substitution for
1 bread, 1 vegetable B, and ½ protein
shares

Chunky Clam Chowder

Exchange Substitution for
1½ protein, 1 vegetable B, and ½ bread
shares

Chunky Chicken with Rice

Exchange Substitution for
1¼ protein, 1 bread, and ½ vegetable B
shares

Chunky Beef

Exchange Substitution for
1¼ protein and 1 bread shares

Chunky Chicken

Exchange Substitution for
1 protein, ½ bread, and ½ vegetable B
shares

Chunky Turkey

Exchange Substitution for
1 vegetable B, ½ bread, and ½ fat
shares

Chunky Vegetable

*1 Cup Portion

Swanson Brand Frozen Prepared Products
Individual Meat Pies
(8 ounces each)

Exchange Substitution for
3 bread, 4 fat, 1 protein, and 1 vegetable B shares

Chicken Pie

Exchange Substitution for
2¼ bread, 4 fat, 1 protein, and 1 vegetable B shares

Turkey Pie

Exchange Substitution for
2 bread, 3 fat, 1½ protein, and 1 vegetable B shares

Beef Pie

Swanson Canned Products *†

Exchange Substitution for
2 protein and 1½ bread shares

Chili Con Carne with Beans

Exchange Substitution for
2 protein, 1 vegetable B, and ½ bread shares

Beef Stew

Exchange Substitution for
1¼ protein, 1 vegetable B, and ½ bread shares

Chicken Stew

Exchange Substitution for
1 protein, ½ bread, and ½ fat shares

Chicken a la King

Exchange Substitution for
1 protein and ½ bread shares

and Beef

*1 Cup Portion

†½ Cup Portion

Deep Dish Meat Pies
(16 ounces each)

Exchange Substitution for
3 bread, 5 fat, 3 protein, and 2
vegetable B shares

Chicken Pie

Exchange Substitution for
3 protein, 3 fat, 2½ bread, and 2
vegetable B shares

Beef Pie
Turkey Pie

"TV" Brand Entrees
(1 complete entree)

Exchange Substitution for
3 protein, 2 bread, and 1½ fat shares

Fried Chicken with Whipped Potatoes

Exchange Substitution for
2 protein, 2 bread, and 1½ fat shares

Salisbury Steak with Crinkle-Cut Potatoes

Exchange Substitution for
2 protein, 1½ fat, 1 bread, and 1 vegetable B shares

Meat Loaf with Tomato Sauce and Whipped Potatoes

Exchange Substitution for
2 protein, 2 bread, and ¼ fat shares

Turkey • Gravy • Dressing with Whipped Potatoes

Exchange Substitution for
2 protein, 1½ bread, 1½ fat, and ½ vegetable B shares

Meatballs with Brown Gravy and Whipped Potatoes

Exchange Substitution for
2 protein, 1½ bread, ½ fat, and ¼ vegetable B shares

Spaghetti in Tomato Sauce with Breaded Veal

**Franco-American
Canned Products***

Exchange Substitution for
2 bread, 1 vegetable B, and ¼ fat shares

Spaghetti in Tomato Sauce with Cheese

Exchange Substitution for
2 bread, ½ fat, and ¼ vegetable B shares

Italian Style Spaghetti in Tomato-
  Cheese Sauce
"SpaghettiOs" in Tomato and
  Cheese Sauce

Exchange Substitution for
1½ bread, 1¼ protein, 1 fat, and ½ vegetable B shares

Spaghetti 'n Beef in Tomato Sauce
Spaghetti with Meatballs in Tomato
  Sauce

Exchange Substitution for
1½ bread, 1¼ protein, and 1 fat shares

Macaroni 'n Beef in Tomato Sauce
"SpaghettiOs" with Sliced
  Franks in Tomato Sauce

Exchange Substitution for
1½ bread, 1½ vegetable B, and 1¼ protein shares

Beef Raviolis in Meat Sauce

Exchange Substitution for
1½ bread, ½ fat, and ½ milk

Macaroni & Cheese

Exchange Substitution for
1¼ bread, 1¼ protein, ½ fat, and ½ vegetable B

"SpaghettiOs" with Little Meatballs in Tomato Sauce

*1 Cup Portion

Q. I love canned tomato soup and canned vegetable soup. If I have a seven-ounce serving of soup, what must I exchange for it?

A. You must substitute one bread share for it.

101

A WEEK OF FIGURE-KEEPER MENUS*

Day One

B		Orange juice
R	**F**	1 soft-boiled egg
E	**A**	1 slice toast
A	**S**	Butter or margarine
K	**T**	1 cup skim milk

Coffee or tea if desired (no more than one tablespoon cream or half & half if desired)

L	One-half cantaloupe filled with ½ cup cottage cheese
U	garnished with seedless grapes
N	1 English muffin, toasted
C	Butter or margarine
H	Coffee or tea if desired with cream as above

D	Bouillon with croutons
I	3 to 4 ounces pork roast with sauerkraut
N	and mushrooms
N	½ cup mashed potatoes
E	Lettuce heart with mayonnaise
R	Baked cinnamon apple, gingersnaps (6 small)
	Coffee or tea if desired with cream as above

S	1 cup skim milk
N	4 Triscuits
A	2 tablespoons peanut butter
C	
K	

*Note: See basic shares lists (pp. 64 through 73) for menu substitutions page.

Day Two

B
R **F**   ½ grapefruit
E **A**   2 5-inch waffles
A **S**   2 tablespoons maple syrup
K **T**   1 teaspoon butter or margarine
            1 cup skim milk
            Coffee or tea if desired (no cream or sugar with this
                luscious breakfast)

L
U   8 ounces Cream of Asparagus Soup (see shares list
N   for soup page 96)
C   One-half sandwich(1 slice bread)
H   3 ounces ham sliced ⅛-inch thick lettuce
           1 teaspoon mayonnaise
       ¾ cup strawberries or 2 halves of canned peaches
       Coffee or tea if desired (1 tablespoon cream or
          half & half if desired)

D
I   4 ounces baked rockfish or halibut with lemon wedge
N   Broiled tomato half
N   Asparagus spears
E   Cabbage slaw
R   Dinner roll with butter or margarine, 1 teaspoon
       1 slice angel food cake
       Coffee or tea if desired (as above)

S   1 cup skim milk
N   1 slice bread
A   1 slice American Cheese ⅛-inch thick. (Toast on
C   one side, turn over, add cheese, run under
K   broiler till golden.)

Day Three

B		1 cup tomato juice
R	**F**	¾ cup puffed wheat with ½ teaspoon sugar
E	**A**	1 slice toast
A	**S**	1 teaspoon butter or margarine
K	**T**	1 cup skim milk
		Coffee or tea if desired (1 tablespoon cream or
		half & half if desired)

L	Tuna (3 ounces)/salad sandwich on two slices bread
U	Carrot curls, radish roses, dill pickle chips
N	1 cup skim milk
C	½ cup orange jello (made with orange jello: 1
H	package,
	1 cup mandarin orange sections)
	Coffee or tea if desired (as above)

D	Swiss steak, 5 ounces
I	Green beans and tiny onions
N	Braised celery
N	Biscuit
E	Tossed salad with low-calorie dressing
R	2 halves canned pears
	Coffee or tea if desired (1 tablespoon cream or
	half & half if desired)

S	1½ cup popped corn
N	2 teaspoons butter
A	
C	
K	

Day Four

B
R F
E A
A S
K T

Orange juice
1 poached egg on
1 slice toast
1 teaspoon butter
1 cup skim milk
Coffee or tea if desired (1 tablespoon cream or
    half & half if desired)

L
U
N
C
H

Hamburger on bun, relish, catsup, however you like
15 potato chips
Lettuce heart with low-calorie dressing
1 apple
Coffee or tea if desired (1 tablespoon cream or
    half & half if desired)

D
I
N
N
E
R

2–3 ounces broiled lamb chops (5 ounces each raw)
Baked potato with 2 tablespoons sour cream
Peas and mushrooms
Pineapple slice on lettuce with mayonnaise
½ cup vanilla ice cream, 2 chocolate chip cookies
Coffee or tea if desired (1 tablespoon cream or
    half & half if desired)

S
N
A
C
K

1 cup skim milk
¾ cup cornflakes
½ teaspoon sugar

Day Five

B		½ cup grapefruit juice
R	**F**	½ cup cooked oatmeal with ½ teaspoon brown sugar
E	**A**	1 slice toast with 1 teaspoon butter or margarine
A	**S**	1 cup skim milk
K	**T**	Coffee or tea if desired (1 tablespoon cream or
		half & half if desired)

L	Franks and beans (2 frankfurters chopped in 1 cup
U	baked beans)
N	1 slice rye bread
C	1 teaspoon butter or margarine
H	Celery sticks
	2 halves canned peaches
	Coffee or tea if desired (1 tablespoon cream or
	half & half if desired)

D	Cocktail (if desired—just a reminder that you can
I	substitute. See list page 73)
N	5 ounces broiled steak
N	Broccoli spears with lemon butter
E	Tossed salad with low-calorie dressing
R	⅛ piece of apple pie (9-inch pie)
	Coffee or tea (1 tablespoon cream or half & half
	if desired)

S	1 cup skim milk
N	2 tablespoons peanut butter
A	1 slice bread
C	
K	

Day Six

B		1 fresh orange, sliced
R	**F**	1 scrambled egg
E	**A**	½ English muffin, toasted
A	**S**	1 teaspoon butter
K	**T**	1 teaspoon your favorite jelly or jam

1 cup skim milk
Coffee or tea if desired (1 tablespoon cream or
   half & half, if desired)

L	7 ounces clam chowder (see soup shares list,
U	page 98) with 1 ounce chopped ham
N	5 saltines
C	Fruit salad on lettuce (1 pear half)
H	(1 peach half)

                 (½ banana, sliced)
1 teaspoon honey dressing
   (see page 108)
Coffee or tea if desired (as above)

D	1 cup spaghetti and 3 1-ounce meatballs plus sauce
I	Tossed salad with Italian tomato dressing
N	(see page 109)
N	Italian bread, 1 slice with teaspoon butter
E	½ cup strawberry or chocolate ice cream
R	Coffee or tea if desired (as above)

S	1 cup skim milk
N	5 round crackers (Ritz)
A	1-inch cube Cheddar cheese (1 ounce)
C	
K	

Recipe for Honey Dressing

¼ cup sugar

1 teaspoon dry mustard

1 teaspoon paprika

1 teaspoon celery seed

¼ teaspoon salt

⅓ cup vinegar

⅓ cup honey

1 tablespoon lemon juice

½ teaspoon grated onion

(You can use all lemon juice in place of vinegar)

In a small mixer bowl mix together sugar, mustard, paprika, celery seed, and salt. Add vinegar, lemon juice, and honey very slowly, beating constantly with rotary or electric beater. Store in refrigerator.

Note: Poppy seeds may be substituted for the celery seed. May be made in blender, but add celery seed by hand. Blender will affect the seeds.

Q. Do you have a good low-calorie Italian dressing to put on my salad?

Make Ahead Italian Tomato Dressing

2 tablespoons oil

⅓ cup cider vinegar

1 (8-ounce) can tomato sauce or puree

½ teaspoon salt

1 teaspoon dry mustard

1 teaspoon paprika

½ teaspoon oregano

2 teaspoons Worcestershire sauce

½ clove garlic, finely chopped

2 teaspoons finely chopped onion

1 tablespoon finely chopped celery

Artificial sweetener to equal 2 tablespoons
sugar—amount depends on your
sweetener—read the label

Combine all ingredients in 1-quart mixing bowl. Beat at medium speed 2 minutes (or blend ingredients in blender for 15 seconds on high speed). Chill. Store in refrigerator; storage time, 1 month. Makes about 1 pint. Although this dressing has a small amount of oil, you can use it without counting it as a fat share since the quantity is small. If the dressing is too tangy or too sweet, you can eliminate both the Worcestershire sauce and sweetener.

Day Seven

B	1 cup tomato juice
R	1 fried egg
E	2 strips crisp bacon
A	1 slice toast
K	½ teaspoon butter or margarine
F	1 cup skim milk
A	Coffee or tea if desired (1 tablespoon cream or
S	half & half if desired)
T	

L	Grilled cheese sandwich
U	Sliced tomatoes on lettuce with low-calorie dressing
N	1 fresh apple
C	Coffee or tea if desired as above, or diet cola
H	

D	½ baked chicken breast
I	½ cup mashed potatoes
N	Peas and carrots
N	Citrus fruit sections on lettuce with low-calorie
E	dressing
R	Dinner roll with ½ teaspoon butter
	1/12 piece of 10-inch chocolate cake
	Coffee or tea if desired (as above)

S	1 cup skim milk
N	5 saltines
A	2 tablespoons peanut butter
C	
K	

Q. I just finished losing twenty-seven pounds and I'm tired of dieting. What shall I do?

A. If you don't think you will stick to a maintenance regimen, it might be a practical plan for you, newly thin, to add new foods in small amounts to be sure no weight gain occurs. Do this until you find your own level—the one at which your weight remains steady. Remember to drink a quart of water a day and to exercise regularly.

4

THE EASY, NO-RISK DIET FOR "CARBOHOLICS"

My medical practice has shown that twelve percent of the people who see me do not handle carbohydrates properly. If this is true of you, then you probably gain an inordinate amount of weight after eating sugar or other carbohydrates.

You might also complain, and rightly so, about being excessively tired, having a fast-racing heart, sweating, feeling weak and anxious, and "not thinking straight" after eating carbohydrates—especially sugar, cookies, candy, cakes, soda pop and ice cream. Often, after eating sweets, you may experience an insatiable desire to continue eating more and more of them. The more you gobble, the more you want—and the worse you feel. The cycle just aggravates your problem. Am I describing you? An abnormal glucose tolerance test (GTT) by your doctor can help substantiate your suspicion that you do not handle carbohydrates normally. I call people with these symptoms "carboholics" and find that they do exceptionally well on my Easy, No-Risk Diet for carboholics. It should be understood that this inability to cope with carbohydrates is not so exaggerated that you have frank hypoglycemia. If you suspect you have hypoglycemia, you should see your doctor who should take a thorough history, do a complete physical examination and order appropriate laboratory tests including a glucose tolerance test. Then, from this information, he can institute appropriate treatment and diet.

THE EASY, NO-RISK DIET FOR CARBOHOLICS

You who have difficulty handling carbohydrates should be able successfully to control weight on this diet. But first check it out with your doctor. He may want to modify it to meet your specific needs. Use my Easy, No-Risk shares lists on pages 64 through 73 with their appropriate servings each day. Note the expanded vegetable list provided in this chapter, and particularly that List 2 must be used for ½ bread share. All other instructions and suggestions for the basic diet are applicable here, including the allowance for an alcoholic beverage three times a week. *The crucial difference is that the carbohydrate, on this version of the diet, drops significantly to about 100 grams—still within nutritionally sound limits.*

You may plan your intake of food any way you wish, but do not exceed the daily 1,200-calorie total amount of food. You may have three meals and a snack or six small meals. For helpful tips on food preparation consult the Cooking Hints for Losing Weight section in Chapter 3 (pages 85 through 88).

EASY, NO-RISK DIET FOR CARBOHOLICS*

EIGHT PROTEIN SHARES

THREE FRUIT SHARES

TWO DAIRY SHARES

THREE FAT SHARES

THREE BREAD SHARES

VEGETABLES—List 1 is free

VEGETABLES—List 2 use as ½ bread share

*1200 calories, 78 grams protein, 57 grams fat, 99 grams carbohydrate

Note: See Master Easy, No-Risk Shares Lists pages 64 through 73 and Carboholics Vegetable Shares Lists page 116.

Vegetable List 1

May be used as desired in ordinary amounts.

Asparagus
Beet Greens
Broccoli
Brussels sprouts
Cabbage (all kinds)
Cauliflower
Celery
Chard
Chicory
Collards
Cucumber
Dandelion greens
Eggplant
Endive
Escarole
Green Beans

Kale
Leeks
Lettuce
Mushrooms
Mustard greens
Okra
Peppers
Poke
Radishes
Sauerkraut
Spinach
Summer squash
Tomatoes
Turnip greens
Watercress
Wax beans

Vegetable List 2

One half cup is to be substituted for ½ bread share.

Beets
Carrots
Kolhrabi
Onions
Oyster plant
Peas (green)

Pumpkin
Rutabagas
Squash (winter)
Turnips
Water chestnuts (7)

NOTE: Vegetables may be raw or cooked in salted water. See hints on low-calorie cooking, pages 87 and 88.

Plan A is a pattern meal for carboholics who *don't* need to watch the number of eggs they eat too closely. Plan B is for egg-watchers. (Also see instructions for controlling cholesterol, pages 89 and 90.)

PATTERN MEAL FOR CARBOHOLICS
(Plan A: For Non-Eggwatchers)

B		1 serving of fruit
R	**F**	1 protein share
E	**A**	1 fat share
A	**S**	1 bread share
K	**T**	½ cup skim milk or buttermilk
		Coffee or tea if desired

L	3 protein shares
U	Vegetables
N	1 fat share
C	1 bread share
H	1 fruit share
	½ cup skim milk or buttermilk
	Coffee or tea if desired

D	3 protein shares
I	Vegetables
N	1 fat share
N	½ cup skim milk or buttermilk
E	1 fruit share
R	Coffee or tea if desired

S	1 protein share
N	1 bread share
A	½ cup skim milk or buttermilk
C	
K	

Note: Snacktime may be as you wish. If your hunger pangs strike in the midafternoon, have it then. Or if the evening is when hunger affects you, snack time should be then. You'll handle carbohydrates better if the intake is spaced throughout the day as this meal plan provides. This is true for either Plan A or B.

PATTERN MEAL FOR CARBOHOLICS
(Plan B: For Eggwatchers)

B		1 serving of fruit	**D**	4 protein shares
R	**F**	2 bread shares	**I**	Vegetables
E	**A**	1 fat share	**N**	1 fat share
A	**S**	1 cup skim milk or buttermilk	**N**	½ cup skim milk or buttermilk
K	**T**	Coffee or tea if desired '	**E**	1 fruit share
			R	Coffee or tea if desired
L		3 protein shares		
U		Vegetables	**S**	1 protein share
N		1 fat share	**N**	1 bread share
C		1 fruit share	**A**	½ cup skim milk or buttermilk
H		Coffee or tea if desired	**C**	
			K	

Note: Snack time may be as you wish. If your hunger pangs strike in midafternoon, have it then. Or if evening is when hunger affects you, plan your snack time then. You'll handle the carbohydrates better if the intake is spaced throughout the day as this meal plan provides.

For your convenience, I have prepared sample menus. Note you have certain freedoms here. If the menu for a meal contains a food you don't like, consult the basic shares lists (pages 64 to 73) and select one you do like. You can interchange fruits, or make substitutions for the bread, or substitute for milk from the dairy list. If the meat does not suit you, select one that does from the protein shares list. Look at the fat shares list for substitutions. Also see expanded vegetable lists on page 116.

The beauty of this diet is its flexibility. You can select foods that are your favorites—forget counting calories. This is done for you.

Note: These seven days menus illustrate different plans of using the daily allowance of food. Use your imagination and vary your intake within the daily limit of food.

FOUR DAYS OF SAMPLE MENUS
FOR CARBOHOLICS
Day One (Plan A: Non-eggwatchers)

B		½ cup orange juice
R	F	1 poached egg on
E	A	1 slice toast with
A	S	1 teaspoon butter or margarine
K	T	½ cup skim milk
		Coffee or tea if desired

L   Tomato stuffed with shrimp salad on lettuce with (15)
U   shrimp, medium size, 2 tablespoons of chopped
N   celery, ½ tablespoon mayonnaise thinned with
C   lemon juice)
H   Cold asparagus spears and pimento slices
     5 saltines
     1 small apple
     Coffee or tea if desired
     ½ cup skim milk or buttermilk

D   ½ pan-broiled chicken breast (use soy sauce
I   to prevent dryness) season with ginger
N   ½ cup lima beans (one bread share) with
N   ½ teaspoon butter or margarine
E   Broiled tomato
R   Tossed salad with low-calorie dressing
     ⅛ honeydew melon or 2 halves of canned peaches,
       water-packed
     Coffee or tea if desired

S   1 cup skim milk or buttermilk
N   1 slice of Cheddar cheese 4 x 4 x ⅛ inches
A   4 Triscuits
C
K

Note: If you don't care for a food, see basic shares lists for menu substitutions (pages 64 through 73 and expanded vegetable lists page 116).

Day Two (Plan A: Non-Eggwatchers)

B
R F
E A
A S
K T

½ cup orange juice
1 egg scrambled (use 1 egg, 1 tablespoon skim milk,
beat and cook in Teflon frying pan, or use
    ½ teaspoon butter or margarine)
½ slice bread, toasted
½ teaspoon butter or margarine
½ cup skim milk minus 1 tablespoon
Coffee or tea if desired

L
U
N
C
H

1 cup bouillon
Broiled open-face sandwich (1 slice bread with 2 slices
    American cheese chopped and 1 slice ham,
    chopped. Mix together, a dash of Tabasco, and
    chopped green pepper. Broil in oven until cheese is
    melted and slightly brown)
Lettuce heart with low-calorie dressing
½ banana
½ cup skim milk or buttermilk
Coffee or tea if desired

D
I
N
N
E
R

1 pan-broiled pork chop
1 small baked potato 2 inches in diameter with
    2 tablespoons sour cream (includes fat share
    from noon) and chives
Green beans with 1 teaspoon butter
Tossed salad—low-calorie dressing
⅓ cup orange sherbet
Coffee or tea if desired

S
N
A
C
K

1 cup skim milk or buttermilk
3 saltines
2 tablespoons peanut butter

Day Three (Plan A: Non-Eggwatchers)

B
R F
E A
A S
K T

1 cup tomato juice
1 coddled egg (place egg in custard cup with 1 tablespoon milk, ½ teaspoon butter, bake in oven or use coddler)
½ teaspoon butter or margarine
1 slice bread, toasted
Coffee or tea as desired

L
U
N
C
H

Oyster stew (made with 1 cup skim milk, 1 teaspoon butter, 6 medium oysters. Cook oysters in liquid from oysters until edges curl, add butter [1 teaspoon], salt to taste and 1 cup skim milk)
2 slices boiled ham
5 saltines
Carrot sticks, celery sticks, and dill pickle sticks
2 halves of canned pears without sugar or 1 fresh pear
Coffee or tea as desired

D
I
N
N
E
R

3 ounces beef cubes in shish kebab—on skewer mushrooms, green pepper, tiny tomatoes
Brush with low-calorie French dressing, broil
Brussels sprouts with 1 tablespoon margarine and lemon juice
Lettuce heart with low-calorie dressing
1 baked apple (medium size) with cinnamon, nutmeg, and artificial sweetener
½ cup skim milk or buttermilk
Coffee or tea if desired

S
N
A
C
K

½ cup skim milk
4 Triscuits or 2 vanilla (Pepperidge Farm) pirouettes

Day Four (Plan A: Non-eggwatchers)

B
R **F**　½ cup grapefruit juice
E **A**　1 egg scrambled (see day two)
A **S**　2 slices crisp bacon
K **T**　1 slice toast, dry
　　　　Coffee or tea if desired

L　　3-ounce hamburger on 1 roll
U　　Dill pickle chips
N　　Tomato slices on lettuce with low-calorie dressing
C　　½ banana
H　　1 cup skim milk or buttermilk
　　　　Coffee or tea if desired

D　　3 ounces broiled ham steak
I　　5-minute cabbage steamed with ½ teaspoon butter or
N　　　　margarine
N　　Green beans with low-calorie dressing
E　　2 halves canned pears without sugar or 1 fresh pear
R　　Coffee or tea if desired

S　　1 cup skim milk
N　　¼ cup cottage cheese
A
C
K

THREE DAYS' SAMPLE MENUS FOR CARBOHOLICS
Day One (Plan B: Eggwatchers)

B
R F
E A
A S
K T

½ cup grapefruit juice
¾ cup cornflakes (remember all cereals must be
   processed without sugar—read labels to be sure
   sugar has not been added)
1 cup skim milk or buttermilk
1 teaspoon butter or margarine
1 slice toast or ½ English muffin
Coffee or tea if desired

L
U
N
C
H

¾ cup cottage cheese or
3 slices cold cuts, 4½ inches square by ⅛ inch thick,
   your favorite, or 3 ounces cold turkey,
   season and wrap in lettuce leaves
Cucumber slices
Lettuce
Dill pickle wedge
2 halves canned peaches, water-packed, or 1 fresh
   peach
Coffee or tea if desired

D
I
N
N
E
R

1 cocktail (see alcohol shares list for exchanges, page
   73) [fat share from noon and P.M.]
4 ounces of broiled steak with broiled mushrooms
Broccoli spears with lemon wedge
½ cup carrot circles with celery
Sliced tomatoes on lettuce with low-calorie dressing
D-Zerta in any flavor, with ½ banana, sliced
Coffee or tea if desired

S
N
A
C
K

1 cup skim milk or buttermilk
½ slice bread or 3 crackers
2 tablespoons peanut butter

*Note: See the basic shares lists for menu substitution pages 64
through 73.

Day Two (Plan B: Eggwatchers)

B R E A K F A S T

1 orange, sliced
½ cup cooked oatmeal
1 cup skim milk or buttermilk
1 teaspoon butter or margarine
1 slice toast
Coffee or tea as desired

L U N C H

1 cup chicken bouillon
¾ cup cottage cheese in tomato on lettuce
Cucumber slices with low-calorie dressing
⅛ honeydew melon or 12 large grapes
Coffee or tea if desired

D I N N E R

2–3 ounces (cooked weight) lamb chops pan broiled
    (5 ounces raw weight)
Parsleyed cauliflower, 1 teaspoon butter or margarine
Spinach with vinegar
Tossed salad with low-calorie dressing
½ broiled grapefruit (put 1 teaspoon butter or margarine on grapefruit half, dash with cinnamon and artificial sweetener. Place under oven broiler until bubbly.)
Coffee or tea if desired

S N A C K

1 cup skim milk or buttermilk
⅛-inch slice luncheon meat
1 slice bread

Day Three (Plan B: Eggwatchers)

B
R F
E A
A S
K T

½ cup orange juice
¾ cup puffed rice
1 cup skimmed milk or buttermilk
1 slice toast or ½ English muffin, toasted
½ teaspoon butter or margarine
Coffee or tea if desired

L
U
N
C
H

Sandwich with 2 slices rye bread
2 ounces lean corned beef
1 slice Swiss cheese
½ cup sauerkraut
toast open faced until cheese melts
top with second slice and eat
1 dill pickle
4 halves canned apricots without sugar or 2 fresh
apricots
Coffee or tea if desired

D
I
N
N
E
R

1 cocktail (2 fat shares)
3-ounce salmon steak, broiled, with low-calorie
dressing
Creole eggplant
Green beans with mushrooms with ½ teaspoon butter
or margarine
½ cup skim milk
12 grapes or ¼ cantaloupe
Coffee or tea if desired

S
N
A
C
K

½ cup skim milk
⅓ cup sherbet
2 graham crackers or 1 sugar cookie 2 inches in
diameter

If you would rather eat six times a day, try this eating style:

Carboholic Meal Plan for Six Meals a Day

B		1 serving fruit
R	**F**	1 protein share
E	**A**	½ bread share
A	**S**	½ fat share
K	**T**	Coffee or tea if desired

M	**M**	½ cup skim milk
I	**O**	½ fat share
D	**R**	½ bread share
	N	
	I	
	N	
	G	

L	2 protein shares
U	1 bread share
N	1 serving List 1 vegetable
C	1 fat share
H	Coffee or tea if desired or diet cola

M	**D**	1 protein share
I	**A**	1 fruit share
D	**Y**	½ cup skim milk

D	3 protein shares
I	2 servings vegetables List 1
N	1 fruit share
N	1 fat share
E	Coffee or tea if desired
R	

S	1 protein share
N	1 bread share
A	½ cup skim milk
C	
K	

After you have reached your ideal weight, follow this maintenance plan to keep slim forever:

FIGURE-KEEPER PLAN FOR THE CARBOHOLIC

To keep your new figure enjoy the following amounts of food every day.

TEN PROTEIN SHARES

THREE FRUIT SHARES

TWO DAIRY SHARES

EIGHT FAT SHARES

THREE BREAD SHARES

VEGETABLES: LIST 1 IS FREE

VEGETABLES: LIST 2—USE ½ BREAD SHARE

(See master Easy, No-Risk Shares Lists pages 64 through 73 and Carboholics Vegetable Shares Lists page 116.)

Two meal plans for maintaining weight loss are listed for your use. Plan I gives you three meals a day and a snack. If you prefer to eat more often, Plan II is suggested, which offers you six feedings a day. Take your choice. You can also switch from Plan I one day to Plan II the next day. Just don't eat both Plan I and Plan II on the same day.

Q. Could you prepare me a seven-day meal plan using Plan I some days and Plan II other days?
A. These are to be used now that you have reached your desired weight. Remember that you must continue to weigh yourself once a week and record weight in your diary. This memory device will help you to take action the moment a weight gain has occurred. It's back on the 1,200-calorie carboholic diet for you until your weight has returned to the desired level. Because of your inability to handle carbohydrates, restrictions on this nutrient will remain.

For amounts of food see basic Shares Lists pages 64 through 73.

FIGURE-KEEPER PLAN FOR THE CARBOHOLIC*

Pattern Meal—Plan I
Three Meals and Snack

B		1 serving fruit
R	**F**	1 protein share
E	**A**	3 fat shares
A	**S**	1 bread share
K	**T**	½ cup skim milk
		Coffee or tea if desired

L	4 protein shares
U	Vegetables, List 1
N	3 fat shares
C	1 bread share
H	1 fruit share
	½ cup skim milk
	Coffee or tea if desired or diet cola

D	4 protein shares
I	Vegetables, List 1
N	3 fat shares
N	1 serving fruit
E	½ cup skim milk
R	Coffee or tea if desired or diet cola

S	1 protein share
N	1 fat share
A	1 bread share
C	½ cup skim milk
K	

*Diet contains 95 grams protein
115 grams fat
99 grams carbohydrate
1,789 calories

129

Pattern Meal Plan II
Six-Feeding Plan

B
R F   1 serving fruit
E A   1 protein share
A S   2 fat shares
K T   ½ bread share
           Coffee or tea if desired

M M   1 fat share
I O   ½ bread share
D R   ½ cup skim milk
N
I
N
G

L   2 protein shares
U   Vegetables, List 1
N   2 fat shares
C   1 bread share
H   ½ fruit share
           Coffee or tea if desired or diet cola

M D   2 protein shares
I A   Vegetables, List 1
D Y   1 fat share
           ½ fruit share
           ½ cup skim milk

D   4 protein shares
I   Vegetables, List 1
N   3 fat shares
N   1 serving fruit
E   Coffee or tea if desired
R

S   1 protein share
N   1 fat share
A   1 bread share
C   1 cup skim milk
K

SEVEN DAYS FIGURE-KEEPER MENUS
FOR CARBOHOLICS

Alternate menus are planned for Pattern Meal Plan I and Pattern Meal Plan II. For persons who are limiting eggs to three per week, use egg substitutes: Eggstra, Cono, Ova-Comp, or Eggbeaters. Follow directions on package for substitution. If you prefer, substitute one protein share for the egg. See shares list, page 64.

Day One (Plan I—Three Meals and a Snack)

B		½ cup orange juice
R	**F**	1 poached egg on 1 slice toast with 1 teaspoon butter
E	**A**	or margarine
A	**S**	½ cup skim milk
K	**T**	Coffee or tea if desired (1 tablespoon cream or
		half & half if desired)

L Cold plate with 2 slices ham, ⅛ inch thick
U   1 slice American cheese, ⅛ inch thick
N   1 slice Swiss cheese, ⅛ inch thick
C   1 fresh tomato cut in wedges
H   3 dill pickle circles

Cold plate with 2 slices ham, ⅛ inch thick
1 slice American cheese, ⅛ inch thick
1 slice Swiss cheese, ⅛ inch thick
1 fresh tomato cut in wedges
3 dill pickle circles
1 teaspoon mayonnaise
½ English muffin toasted with 1 teaspoon butter or margarine
1 fresh pear or 12 grapes
½ cup skim milk
Coffee or tea if desired (as above), or diet cola

D *Cocktail
I 5 ounces broiled sirloin steak
N French cut green beans with 1 teaspoon butter or
N margarine
E Parsley cauliflower with 1 teaspoon butter or
R margarine
Tossed green salad with low-cal dressing
½ cup pineapple, fresh or water-packed
Coffee or tea if desired (as above)

S 1 cup skim milk
N 1 soft pretzel with 1 teaspoon butter or margarine and
A mustard
C
K

*See drinks list page 73 if you wish to substitute fat shares for a before-dinner drink.

Day Two (Plan II—Six Feeding)

You may find that you feel better with six small meals daily. To show you how to space your food throughout the day, six meals are shown on alternate days.

B		½ cup grapefruit juice
R	**F**	1 egg, soft-boiled
E	**A**	1 teaspoon butter or margarine
A	**S**	½ slice toast
K	**T**	Coffee or tea if desired (1 tablespoon cream, or half & half if desired)

M	**M**	½ cup skim milk
I	**O**	½ toasted English muffin
D	**R**	1 teaspoon butter or margarine
	N	
	I	
	N	
	G	

	Salad—½ cup tuna fish
	2 tablespoons chopped celery
L	2 tablespoons chopped green pepper
U	mix with low-calorie dressing
N	5 medium green olives
C	4 Triscuits
H	D-Zerta with ¾ cup mandarin orange sections water-packed
	Coffee or tea if desired (as above)

M	**D**	½ cup cottage cheese on lettuce
I	**A**	Asparagus spears with 1 teaspoon mayonnaise
D	**Y**	½ cup skim milk
		½ cup strawberries or ½ orange
		Diet cola if desired

D			*Cocktail
I			½ pan-broiled chicken breast
N			Broccoli spears with lemon butter (1 teaspoon)
N			Lettuce heart with 2 teaspoons French dressing
E			2 halves peaches water-packed or fresh
R			Coffee or tea if desired (as above)
B	**T**	**S**	1 cup skim milk
E	**I**	**N**	1 slice ham ⅛ inch thick
D	**M**	**A**	1 slice rye bread with 1 teaspoon butter or margarine
	E	**C**	or mayonnaise
		K	lettuce
			mustard if desired

*See drink list page 73 if you wish to substitute fat shares for a before-dinner drink.

Day Three (Plan I—Three Meals and Snack)

B R E A K **F A S T**

½ cup orange juice
¾ cup cornflakes
½ cup skim milk with 2 tablespoons light cream
Coffee or tea if desired

L U N C H

3 ounces grilled beef patty on
    ½ hamburger bun with 1 slice American cheese
    1 slice tomato
    1 slice onion
Broiled till cheese melts
Coleslaw with 3 teaspoons mayonnaise
⅛ honeydew melon or 1 small apple
½ cup skim milk
Coffee or tea if desired

D I N N E R

Cocktail—2 fat shares—one from A.M. and one from
    P.M.
5 clams, broiled. (Place five fresh clams on shells, put
    1 drop Tabasco sauce on each, put 1 tiny piece of
    tomato, either canned or fresh on each clam, chop
    ½ slice bacon [½ fat exchange] sprinkle on clams.
    Place under broiler and cook until bacon is crisp.
    Delicious with your cocktail).
3 ounces baked ham
Wax beans with 1 teaspoon butter or margarine
Spinach with ½ teaspoon butter or margarine
Tossed salad with low-calorie dressing
2 halves canned pears, water-packed, or 1 fresh pear
Coffee or tea if desired

S N A C K

1 cup skim milk
Fried egg sandwich
    1 egg fried in 1 teaspoon butter or margarine
    1 slice bread

Day Four (Plan II—Six Feedings)

B
R F
E A
A S
K T

½ grapefruit
1-ounce wedge of cheese (your favorite)
1 teaspoon butter or margarine
½ toasted English muffin
Coffee or tea if desired

A.
M.

½ cup skim milk
2 honey graham crackers
1 teaspoon butter or margarine

L
U
N
C
H

½ sandwich made with (1 slice bread, 2 slices of
    your favorite luncheon meat or cheese or a mixture
    of both, 1 teaspoon mayonnaise or margarine lettuce
    leaf
Celery curls
Cucumber slices
6 grapes or ⅛ cantaloupe
Diet cola or coffee or tea if desired

M D
I A
D Y

2 slices luncheon meat
Tomato slices—1 teaspoon mayonnaise
6 grapes or ⅛ cantaloupe
½ cup skim milk

D
I
N
N
E
R

Cocktail (2 fat shares 1 A.M. and 1 noon)
2–4 ounce pork chops pan broiled
Sauerkraut or 7-minute cabbage—1 teaspoon butter or
    margarine
Green beans with 1 teaspoon butter or margarine
Waldorf salad: 1 small apple diced with skin on
               1 tablespoon chopped celery
               6 pecan halves chopped
               mix with low-calorie dressing,
                 serve on lettuce
Coffee or tea if desired

S
N
A
C
K

1 cup skim milk
2 tablespoons peanut butter on
    either 5 saltines or 1 slice bread
1 teaspoon butter

Day Five (Plan I—Three Meals and a Snack)

B R E A K F A S T

1 cup fresh strawberries or ½ cup orange juice
1 poached egg on 1 slice toast, 1 teaspoon butter or margarine
½ cup skim milk
Coffee or tea if desired

L U N C H

Cold plate: ½ cup cottage cheese
2 slices luncheon meat ⅛ inch thick
½ avocado (4 inches in diameter) sliced
½ grapefruit sectioned—alternate with
avocado slices
on lettuce with low-calorie dressing if
desired
3 Rye Krisp
½ cup skim milk
Coffee or tea if desired, or diet cola

D I N N E R

4 ounces filet of flounder, broiled, spread with 2
teaspoons mayonnaise, dash paprika
Asparagus spears with 1 teaspoon margarine or butter
Broiled half tomato with 1 teaspoon margarine or
butter
Tossed green salad with low-calorie dressing
Two halves peaches water-packed, or fresh peach
Coffee or tea if desired

S N A C K

1 cup skim milk
3 sardines
5 round crackers

137

Day Six (Plan II—Six Feedings)

B		½ cup orange juice
R	**F**	1 egg, soft-boiled
E	**A**	1 teaspoon butter or margarine
A	**S**	½ slice bread, toasted
K	**T**	Coffee or tea if desired

A.   ½ cup skim milk
M. 1 teaspoon butter or margarine
One-half of a ½-inch slice pound cake, toasted

L 2 frankfurters, broiled
U   mustard if you wish
N Broccoli spears with 1 teaspoon butter or margarine
C 1 slice rye bread
H 1 teaspoon butter or margarine
    ½ apple
    Coffee or tea if desired, or diet cola

P. 10 small shrimp with 1 teaspoon mayonnaise
M. Relishes—pickle strips (dill)
          celery sticks
          green pepper strips
    ½ apple
    ½ cup skim milk

D 2–4 ounce lamb chops pan broiled (6 ounces raw
I   weight)
N Brussels sprouts with 1 teaspoon butter or margarine
N Tossed salad with 2 teaspoons French dressing
E D-Zerta with ½ banana
R Coffee or tea if desired

S 1 cup skim milk
N 1 slice luncheon meat
A 1 slice bread
C 1 teaspoon butter or margarine
K

Note: If cocktail is desired, some of the fat from evening and midmorning or afternoon could be used. It is important to keep the milk and bread shares divided as in the meal plan. Fat shares may be used however you wish.

Day Seven (Plan I—Three-Meal Plan and a Snack)

B R E A K F A S T

½ grapefruit
1 scrambled egg with 1 tablespoon cream
1 strip of bacon, fried crisp
1 slice toast
1 teaspoon butter or margarine
½ cup skim milk
Coffee or tea if desired

L U N C H

1 sandwich: 2 slices bread
            4 slices of cheese or luncheon meat ⅛ inch thick
            sliced tomato
            1 teaspoon butter or margarine
            lettuce leaf, dill pickle slices
Tossed salad with 2 teaspoons French dressing or mayonnaise
4 halves canned apricots water-packed or 2 fresh
½ cup skim milk
Coffee or tea if desired, or diet cola

D I N N E R

Cocktail (2 fat shares)
5 ounces roast beef
Cauliflower with tomato with ½ teaspoon butter or margarine
Summer squash with ½ teaspoon butter or margarine
Lettuce heart with low-calorie dressing
Watermelon without rind (1 cup) or 12 Royal Anne cherries, water-packed
Coffee or tea if desired

S N A C K

1 cup skim milk
1½ cups popped corn with 1 teaspoon butter

If you are a newly thin carboholic, you may not want to go on another diet right away to maintain your weight. If so, just add new food in small amounts, to be sure no weight gain occurs, until you find your own level at which your weight remains stable.

5

THE MINIDIET—

FOR WORKING PEOPLE

WHO WON'T TAKE

TIME TO

DIET

This is a minichapter which gives you a minidiet. It is especially for newspaper reporters, crooks, politicians, actresses, television directors, dog trainers, schoolteachers, businessmen, businesswomen, young doctors, students, moonlighters, authors, and anyone else who leads a hectic, unstructured life.

You're fat. You know you are. You don't like it. But you just don't have time to spend concentrating on exactly what amount of which foods you should be eating. You never know from one day to the next what hour you're going to be eating, and consider yourself lucky that you get to eat at all.

You've tried some diets, but the monotony and boredom turned you off.

You know perfectly well you are not going to stick to any diet—no matter how promising its variety—because other things take precedence in your life. And you're just not going to take the time to prepare a special diet.

You take what you do seriously. So—when it comes to dieting—don't kid yourself. If you won't spend the necessary time going on my safe, easy, no-risk diet, then don't even try it. Instead, try this very simple minidiet.

Make three copies of the minidiet on file cards for your pocket or purse, the office, your home.

Check with your doctor before you go on this or any diet. He may want to modify it to meet your particular needs. You do not need to take any vitamin or mineral supplements while on this minidiet, because the diet provides you with all the nutrients you need to stay well—yet, it will result in a gradual weight loss if faithfully followed. If you have a medical problem that necessitates your taking vitamins, you should consult your doctor.

There are only three simple rules to follow on the Minidiet:

Rule No. 1: Drink a glass of water before each meal.

Rule No. 2: Don't eat anything that is not on the following menus.

Rule No. 3: If you want to drink alcohol have no more than one drink every third day. Go to our alcohol list on page 73. Do not subtract anything from this diet without first consulting your physician.

MINIDIET *

Breakfast

Fruit or fruit juice, 4 ounces
Bread, 1 slice
1 pat of butter or margarine; or 1 slice of crisp bacon; or 2
tablespoons of light cream or 1 fat share
Egg—1 soft-boiled, poached, or fried in Pam or substitute 1 ounce
lean meat, fish, or poultry or cheese.
Or 1 serving of cereal† (hot or cold)
Skimmed milk, 1 cup

Lunch

Lean meat, chicken or fish, 3 ounces
1 cooked vegetable, average serving, and green salad with
low-calorie dressing
Fruit, fresh in season
1 slice of bread; or 1 roll; or ½ bagel or 1 bread share

Dinner

Lean meat, chicken or fish, 4 ounces
2 cooked vegetables or 1, plus a green salad with low-calorie
dressing
1 slice of bread; or 1 roll; or ½ bagel; or 1 bread share
Fresh fruit, low-calorie pudding or ½ cup jello (average serving)

Snack or Bedtime
1 cup skim milk

*Contains approximately 1,200 calories, 83 grams protein, 47 grams fat, 113 grams carbohydrate.

†Avoid cereals prepared with dried fruits, sugar, honey, coconut, or nuts. (Note: For variation, you can scramble the egg using some of the milk; also you can use your milk with the cereal.)

You may also have limited tea or coffee or water as you desire. In addition you may have up to three 8-ounce glasses of diet or club soda a day. You may also have one cup of beef or chicken broth each day.

Include a food rich in vitamin C each day such as citrus fruits, cantaloupe, strawberries, tomatoes, or tomato juice. Cabbage, Brussels sprouts, greens, such as spinach, kale, mustard greens, and potatoes cooked in their skins are also rich sources.

That is the amount of food allowed for the day. But you can make substitutions. You can substitute from within the basic, Easy, No-Risk Diet Shares lists (Chapter 3, pages 64 through 73.)

As important as what you eat is what you don't eat. Except for every third day, AVOID alcohol, beer, and wine. Also avoid jam, jelly, peanut butter, candy, soda pop, nuts, ice cream (except as allowed), cream soup made with milk, sausage, pancakes, waffles, all sauces, fried foods, cereal already sweetened, and bought baked goods.

(Tips: Cut all the fat from meats. Bake, boil, or broil meat, fish, poultry. Stay out of bakeries. Make your own low-calorie goodies.)

SAMPLE MENUS FOR THE MINIDIET

These menus are planned for the busy individual whose consuming passion is career. The noon meal is expected to be eaten out or carried in a brown bag. These menus contain the day's total amount of food. Do not interchange these menus.

Day One

Breakfast   ½ cup orange juice
in a jiffy   1 egg poached on 1 slice toast with 1 teaspoon
butter or margarine
1 cup skimmed milk
Coffee or tea if desired

Lunch   Cheeseburger—one 2-ounce beef patty (usual
size) with 1 slice cheese
1 bun
Dill pickle slices
Tossed vegetable salad with low-calorie dressing.
(If not available at your favorite fast-food place, ask for lemon
wedge, use juice from it and salt and pepper on salad
12 grapes in plastic bag or apple from home
Coffee or tea if desired or low-calorie cola

Dinner   4 ounces roast beef (3 × 4 × ¼ inches thick)
Broccoli spears cooked in bouillon with lemon
wedge
Carrot rings with parsley
Lettuce heart with low-calorie dressing
D-Zerta with ½ cup water-packed fruit cocktail (or
just the fruit cocktail)
or ½ cup vanilla ice cream
Coffee or tea if desired

Snack   1 cup skim milk

Day Two

Breakfast 1 cup tomato juice
¾ cup cornflakes
1 cup skim milk or ½ cup whole milk
Coffee or tea if desired

Lunch Brown bagging it:
¾ cup cottage cheese (keep cool in a wide-mouthed thermos) or 3 slices (3 ounces) turkey breast (your delicatessen is a good source)
Relishes—celery sticks, carrot sticks, radish roses, lettuce
7 round crackers—Ritz for example, or 1 slice bread
1 fresh orange
Coffee or tea if desired, or diet cola

Dinner Seafood platter—15 steamed shrimp with Dippy Dressing*
½ cup crab meat or water-packed tuna, lemon wedge
Asparagus spears
Steamed summer squash
Tomato wedges and cucumber slices on lettuce
2 halves of water-packed peaches or 1 fresh peach in season or ½ banana
Coffee or tea if desired, or diet cola

Snack 1 cup skim milk
4 Triscuits
1 slice American cheese ⅛ inch thick

Dippy Dressing (1 teaspoon low-calorie dressing, 1 teaspoon mayonnaise, 1 teaspoon pickle relish, ½ teaspoon onions chopped, 1 teaspoon catsup)

146

Day Three

Breakfast ½ cup orange juice
1 soft-boiled egg
1 slice toast with ½ teaspoon butter or margarine
Coffee or tea if desired

Lunch Sandwich with 2 slices rye bread
2 slices ham ⅛ inch thick
1 slice American cheese
slice tomato
lettuce
1 medium-sized apple or 1 pear
1 cup skimmed milk
Coffee or tea if desired

Dinner 1 cup beef or chicken bouillon
½ half oven-broiled or pan-fried chicken breast
Creole eggplant: eggplant simmered with tomato,
green pepper, celery, using only ½ teaspoon
butter or margarine as seasoning
Green beans
Tossed green salad with low-calorie dressing
¼ cantaloupe or ¾ cup strawberries or ½
grapefruit
Coffee or tea if desired

Snack 1 cup skim milk

Notice you can have a drink mixed with club soda or water every third day. Choose one of the following: 1½ ounces scotch, bourbon, rye, gin, rum or vodka—1 glass (3½ ounces) of dry red wine or white wine, or domestic sherry.

If you follow my Minidiet and get an average amount of exercise, you will lose weight.

Q. **How can I control the weight loss achieved by the Minidiet?**

A. Weigh yourself undressed once a week at approximately the same time of day. This way you can detect weight gain before it becomes a problem. If you're gaining, it's back on the diet. It's a good idea to keep a written diary. For maintenance simply follow the Minidiet Figure-Keeper Plan. If you gain weight, go back to the Minidiet until you lose again.

MINIDIET FIGURE-KEEPER PLAN *

Breakfast

Fruit or fruit juice, 6 ounces
Bread, 2 slices
2 pats of butter or margarine or 2 slices of crisp bacon, or 2 fat
  shares
Egg—1 soft-boiled, poached or fried in Pam or substitute 1 ounce
  lean meat, fish, poultry or cheese.
Or 1 serving cereal† (hot or cold)
Skimmed milk, 1 cup, or 1 cup whole milk

Lunch

3 ounces lean meat, chicken, or fish
1 cooked vegetable, average serving and green salad with
  low-calorie dressing
Fruit, fresh in season
2 slices bread or 2 rolls or 1 bagel or 2 bread shares
1 fat share

Dinner

Lean meat, chicken, or fish, 5 ounces
2 cooked vegetables or 1 cooked vegetable and salad with
  low-calorie dressing
2 slices bread or 2 bread shares
Fruit (fresh or canned), pudding ½ cup, jello ½ cup, ½ cup ice
  cream
1 or 2 fat shares

Snack

1 cup milk
1 slice or 1 bread share
1 fat share

*Contains approximately 1600–1900 calories, 95 grams protein, 70–90 grams fat, 175 grams carbohydrate.
†Avoid cereals prepared with dried fruits, sugar, honey, coconut or nuts. (Note: For variation, you can scramble the egg using some of the milk; also, you can use your milk with the cereal.)

6

DIET

MEDITATION ("DM")—

HOW TO STAY ON

YOUR DIET

I have failed on every diet in the past. Why will I be successful on this one?

Because I'm going to change your attitude and you're going to help me do it. And because this is a *nutritionally sound, painless, easy-to-follow diet that gives you all the vitamins and minerals that your body needs for optimal function.* You'll feel good about the diet, and you'll actually feel good. I will give you a new approach to dieting that will allow you to stay on the diet and lose weight successfully.

DIET MEDITATION—"DM"

● Psyche up your subconscious through a simple process called *affirmative automatic response.* Since your subconscious now chiefly knows past dietary failures, you will alter it so that it anticipates dietary success and, from that point on, things you do subconsciously will be directed at making you a successful dieter.

• Increase your willpower through *positive suggestion.* Then, once you start dieting, your willpower will be constantly strengthened, because you will continually look and feel better. And that will be the stimulus to greater willpower—greater weight loss—and to looking and feeling even better. Your success will snowball dramatically. Look better—lose weight—look better—lose more weight.

• Keep a *daily diary* (described on page 157) and see exactly where you went off your diet and then remedy any lapses by modifying your behavior with *corrective action.*

Maximum success will be accomplished by using all three techniques. It really is very easy.

Affirmative automatic response—the main thing here is to get your subconscious mind to *know* that you will be successful with your dieting. Then all subconscious action will be automatic and help you succeed.

Dorothy, a thirty-seven-year-old housewife with two teen-age children, lives in the Bronx, and works part-time as a lingerie saleslady in a major New York City department store. She is once-divorced but now happily remarried. She is fifteen pounds over her ideal weight, and has been on many diets and has failed on all of them.

Dorothy went on our Easy, No-Risk Diet and lost four pounds during the first week. Then she dined out at an excellent Italian restaurant that specialized in tempting, fattening, highly spiced and seasoned food. That single lapse meant a three-pound weight gain. Subconsciously, Dorothy must have said, "It's no use—I dieted for a week, lost four pounds, ate one meal and gained three pounds—it just isn't worth it. I'm a diet disaster and am doomed to failure." Subconsciously Dorothy had remembered all the past diets when she had lost weight temporarily, then gained it back as soon as she stopped dieting. Because of this subconscious failure attitude and the "diet-be-damned" attitude, she went off the diet with a vengeance, eating indiscriminately for the next two weeks and gaining twelve pounds.

Though Dorothy's subconscious was now geared for failure, I managed to convince her to master *Diet Meditation*—the new psychological approach. She went back on our diet, was doing very well, and had lost five pounds in two weeks. Then she confronted a similar situation. She was again invited out to dinner. But this time she handled the situation very differently. Subconsciously, her signals did not allow her to return to the Italian restaurant that had been her downfall. Instead, she selected one that served food consistent with her diet.

Q. How do you program your subconscious for dietary success rather than failure?

A. This is Diet Meditation, with its emphasis on affirmative automatic response. To achieve this state you first feed into your subconscious the right information. Follow these five steps:

● Every morning when you get up and every evening before you retire, sit or lie down and get as comfortable as possible. This will be your daily Diet Meditation period. Put everything out of your mind except pleasant thoughts. It doesn't matter what they are, just as long as they are comforting to you. The first step is to be entirely comfortable.

- Simply close your eyes—not tightly, but comfortably.
- Picture in your mind something relaxing—anything that relaxes you. It might be a beautiful sunset or a quiet moment in the country or a time alone with someone you love and love to be with. Whatever relaxes you. So far, these three steps should take less than one minute. Now you are ready for step 4.
- With your eyes closed, relaxing with this comfortable picture in your mind, slowly count backward from 9 to 1. After each number take a deep breath through your nostrils, holding it for a few seconds and then blowing it out again through your nose. With each countdown and deep breath you will relax additionally. Don't speak to yourself. Practice this breathing technique until you have it down pat, so that you will not have to think about what you're actually doing when you do it. The whole secret is being comfortable and getting progressively more relaxed each time you count backward from 9. By the time you have counted to 1, and have taken nine deep breaths in and out, *you are totally relaxed.* You are now ready for step 5.
- Project in your mind's eye (concentrate on the back of your eyelids) a picture of how you would like to look when you are nice and thin. See how attractive you look with your new figure. You are now a thin person. Now, as this thin person, picture what you would enjoy doing most— whatever it is, no inhibitions, whatever you would most thoroughly enjoy doing as this new, thin person. Finally, picture in your mind's eye how you will solve a particular eating problem without giving in to temptation. That is, experience this mental picture solution *as the new thin you.* The last thought you should have in your mind is that, when you open your eyes, you will feel very relaxed and be

153

able to follow through on your diet completely. This whole procedure should last no more than five minutes. Do this as soon as you get up every morning and before you go to bed every night.

Let's go back to Dorothy and her pasta lapse. Because after the weight gain she felt discouraged and went completely off her diet, Dorothy followed my instructions carefully. She set her alarm clock fifteen minutes earlier in the morning so that she could go through Diet Meditation without being rushed or hassled. She also told her husband what she was doing so he wouldn't interrupt or make fun of her. She had practiced the technique of breathing and counting backward from 9 so she didn't have to think consciously about how long she would hold her breath or how slowly to count. She automatically knew what to do.

She had found that lying flat in bed on her back, with a pillow under her head, was the most comfortable position for her. She had also determined what scene she would project to relax herself—a beach scene. She found a photograph taken when she was very slender and which she liked very much. After studying it she pictured in her mind how she would *like* to look. The photograph was actually taken at the time of her second wedding, when Dorothy was at her ideal weight of 105 pounds. Being exactly five feet tall, she looked marvelous. During DM she perceived herself as a new, thin person and the thing she wanted most to do was to have sex with her husband on a private beach at twilight.

Dorothy had also decided in advance that the problem she would solve during this positive-suggestion period would be the restaurant lapse with the subsequent weight gain and abandonment of her diet. The solution would be to choose a restaurant that focused not just on tempting, fattening, thoroughly spiced foods, but featured, as well, an array of simple but well-prepared chicken, chops, steaks, veal, or seafood.

This way she would avoid the inordinate weight gain, which was partly fluid anyway, and would find it easier to follow her diet. Having thought these things through, she then followed the five simple steps and had a thoroughly enjoyable experience. The last thought she projected in her mind was that when she opened her eyes she would feel very relaxed and would be able to follow her diet completely.

For her positive-suggestion period in the evening, Dorothy altered the mental picture considerably: Her relaxing scene was the deep blue sky. She kept the same new, slender image of herself drawn from the photo, but her objective was different. The thing she most enjoyed doing was being on the beach, surrounded by many men who were vying for her attention. As each man came near, he would eye her admiringly. And why not? She was a beautiful lady with a beautiful body.

In her evening Diet Meditation, Dorothy chose to solve the problem of her persistent desire for sweets. Her solution was to substitute a sour pickle for the sweets, or some sweet she had set aside from her daily shares, which would satisfy her sweet craving and, at the same time, was allowed on her diet. Each day Dorothy had new, relaxing thoughts and solved new problems. Sometimes she reinforced her positive diet attitude, solving the old problems with the same solutions. The one constant was the mental picture of the "new" Dorothy—trim, slim, and perpetually appealing. During the problem-solving, the important thing was coming up with a positive solution to the problem—not berating herself, and *never* giving in to temptation.

Dorothy had never before had the willpower to resist a conscious temptation to eat candy—piece after piece of chocolate would vanish once she got started, until it was all consumed. But now, through willpower enhanced by daily Diet Meditation, she was able to eat a pickle instead, or some other sweet saved from her daily shares. And, she was satisfied, because in her mental solution to the problem, she had been *satisfied* by this instead of candy.

So far it sounds pretty easy, doesn't it? But sometimes problems that you didn't anticipate arise during the day.

When this happened, and Dorothy felt she was about to surrender to temptation, she would simply go through an additional five-minute input of affirmative automatic response—thinking through a practical solution to the particular craving she faced. She would eat a cube of heartily flavored Cheddar and a cracker, or a navel orange, oozing juice, instead of the sweet.

About two months into Diet Meditation, Dorothy discovered she was able to get reinforcement simply by looking into a mirror and smiling. While gazing at herself in the mirror she would reinforce her affirmative automatic response. This generalized reinforcement technique is helpful, if you don't have a specific and immediate temptation problem to solve. It works by reinforcing the overall positive input into your subconscious.

Very important: The positive suggestion of affirmative automatic response can strengthen your willpower. Dorothy had never had the willpower to stay on a diet before practicing diet meditation. Now she possesses it. The times she lapses are when she gives in to old habits. For instance, every time Dorothy's husband, a traveling salesman, was away from home for more than two weeks, Dorothy gained four to ten pounds. She had no idea why. Since she didn't understand the specific problem, she could not mentally program a solution into her subconscious. To get around this new stalemate, I tried a variation of behavior modification used by Dr. Albert Stunkard at Stanford University. I call this *Corrective Action.*

I had Dorothy keep a diary during the first week of her husband's absence. She was self-conscious about carrying the recommended small spiral notebook, so she used instead a single 8½ × 11 inch sheet of paper, folded so that it fitted easily into her purse or into a pocket. She had five columns written across the top: 1. *Time*—that is, the exact time she ate. 2. *Type of food or drink*—that is, exactly what she ate or drank and how much. 3. *Place of eating or drinking*—the exact location where it took place. 4. *Company*—Did she eat by herself or with someone; if so, with whom? 5. *Inner feelings*—What was her state of mind when she ate? Was she bored, tired, troubled, frustrated (sexually or otherwise), depressed, or what?

It was remarkable. A clear-cut pattern quickly developed. Dorothy saw that three days after her husband left, she started to use sweets—candy, cookies, cakes, Cokes. And she ate or drank them at the same time every evening: during the period from half an hour after dinner until she went to bed. The place was at home, and when she ate she always experienced the same feeling—she was lonesome for her husband. She then realized that she bought these delicacies at a confectionery store she passed on her way home from the subway stop after work. So she used a combination of affirmative automatic response and corrective action techniques to help resolve the problem.

First, in her Diet Meditation period she mentally programmed a solution. Then she actually did take an alternate route home so she did not pass the confectionery store. She next dealt with the problem of the loneliness gap. Anticipating it, she arranged ahead to have dinner with friends, see an early movie, or participate in some activity. This way she had something to look forward to that would fill her time. Or she bought a book she had been wanting to read for a long time or borrowed one from the library. On other evenings the solution was doing some of her paperwork at night or watching a special TV show. She also arranged to speak to her husband at a predetermined time each night. When she still felt the urge to eat, she ate instead of sweets the dietary items she had previously prepared and kept in her refrigerator—raw vegetables, carrots, celery stalks, green peppers—and she drank a lot of water and diet soda. She tried to keep food temptations out of the house during these dangerous times.

This, then, is corrective action—Dorothy's determining her pattern, seeing where she went off the diet by eating junk sweets, and then altering her behavior patterns to solve the problem. Once the pattern of compulsive eating is recognized, a combination of affirmative automatic response, positive suggestion, and corrective action is the answer to successful dieting.

The Iceberg Phenomenon

Dieting is a team effort. It takes your conscious and your subconscious working together, cheered on by your will-power I call this the "iceberg phenomenon."

Only a small amount of what you do is conscious behavior—visible above the water like the top of an iceberg. The balance of the iceberg lies under the surface, and that's where affirmative automatic response comes into play. You are doing things you are not aware of. You are doing them automatically.

Remember—your subconscious has no ability to reason, no ability to initiate change. It will only do what it's been programmed to do. Therefore, it is terribly important that the part of the iceberg under the water gets properly programmed so that your mind is constantly geared for successful dieting. Diet Meditation does work, and it can work for you if you believe in it and follow it.

USE A PRACTICAL SOLUTION

Elizabeth, who lives in Albuquerque, sells office furniture. She was fifty-one and fourteen pounds overweight. She went on our diet and lost the excess pounds in six weeks. Elizabeth does well dieting, except when she stops off at the supermarket on her way home from work and buys a lot of things that look tempting at the end of a stressful day. Once she gets home, she quickly realizes that she has overbought. She rationalizes that she now feels obliged to *use* these foods since she has them in her cupboard.

The answer is: Don't go to the supermarket when you're hungry. And when you do go, don't loiter in the cake and pastry aisles. Remember, it's much easier to say no in the supermarket than no at home. When Elizabeth realized this, she planned her menus ahead and bought only the ingredients she needed. Her list did *not* include those nonessential goodies not on her diet. She still had to shop on her way home, but she saved some fruit from lunch and ate it late in the afternoon. This way she did not have to go to the store frantically hungry. She no longer had the overbuy problem, which had caused her home overstock problem, which in turn had added up to her overweight problem.

BE YOUR OWN BOSS

Q. How do you resist the promptings of friends and family who say, "Take a second serving" or "Just taste a little bit of this" or "How drawn you look since you lost weight—you should start eating again" or "Oh, my goodness, it looks like you've lost all your weight from your face and bust"?

A. Alice, a housekeeper from El Paso, fifty-two years young, with fiery red hair, has learned how to handle the situation effectively and diplomatically. She tells her friends and family that she is going on the diet and would like their help. Their contribution to her effort, she advises them, is this: If they don't have anything positive to say, refrain from comment and offer her no seconds. If they start being critical directly or indirectly, she immediately stops them and says, "I am doing this according to my doctor's orders." Alice lost her nineteen excess pounds in seven weeks on our Easy, No-Risk Diet.

BE TRUE TO YOURSELF

Don't wolf your food. Some patients tell me they have to rush to eat because of work pressures or family chores—but that then they never feel quite full.

Barbara, a fifty-year-old men's and boys' apparel saleslady from Milwaukee, had this problem. She used to eat quickly. But then she learned that you should spend twenty minutes eating each meal because it takes twenty minutes after you eat for your stomach to expand enough to signal the brain that you have had enough.

If you are through eating before the twenty minutes, the signal may never get up to the brain. Remember, your stomach is twenty minutes ahead of your brain when it comes to feeling satisfied after eating.

Q. It's a job to spend twenty minutes eating. I am always through in less than ten. How can I possibly extend my eating time to twenty minutes per meal?

A. If you normally eat fast, put your fork or spoon down after each taste of food and chew the food slowly. Relish each morsel, then pick the silverware up again. That should simultaneously increase the enjoyment and the amount of time you spend eating.

Make a conscious effort to spend twenty minutes at

your meals—not including the time it takes to order or prepare them. If dinnertime has previously been a time for airing family gripes and solving problems, alter the routine. Set a specific non-mealtime for family meetings. Strive, if you're eating with a friend or with the family, to make meals a calm, conversational time. Make it a rule, if necessary, that problems are to be left at the dining room door.

7

SUCCESSFUL
DIETERS
SHARE THEIR
SECRETS

DIETERS LOVE COMPANY

"You know Alcoholics Anonymous? I wish there were something like that for people who are overweight," a sixteen-year-old patient of mine said wistfully. Terry had lost sixty-five pounds steadily during the eleven months that followed her first visit to me. But now she was still twenty pounds overweight and getting stronger and stronger urges to go off her diet.

Terry feels her problems are very, very personal. She says she doesn't have many close friends, wonders if she'll ever have a date, and is unhappy at home. She realizes that emotional crises bring on her almost overwhelming impulses to eat large quantities of such junk-food favorites as pizza, potato chips, pretzels, and more nutritional but still fattening ice cream. It is at these moments, when her willpower is most severely strained, that she would like to be able to dial a number and have someone talk her out of her food binge.

Being alone and upset or depressed is a crisis in itself. If you're fat and your inclination is to reach for food to soothe and comfort yourself, it's even more painful. It *does* help to talk. Some successful dieters say they are able actually to talk *themselves* out of a craving for some favorite nondiet delectable. If you can't do that, call a sympathetic friend, or take a walk, or immerse yourself in some activity so that you forget you ever wanted to eat. If you do get as far as the refrigerator door, just make sure it's a carrot, celery stick, sour pickle, low-calorie dessert, or something else allowed on your diet that you pop into your mouth.

Because people do need each other in times of stress, many dieters find diet clubs a big help. At weekly meetings with others who share the same problem, they find a sort of group therapy. And diet-club leaders and instructors who have been through what members are experiencing, and have made it, and keep making it, can be a dramatic inspiration. Many people who did extremely well on our Easy, No-Risk Diet or our Easy, No-Risk Diet for Carboholics did so while simultaneously attending one of the diet clubs. Although they used my diet, they liked the support and camaraderie of the diet club.

The three internationally known diet clubs are Weight Watchers, Diet Workshop, and TOPS (Take Off Pounds Sensibly). TOPS is a nonprofit association. The other two are not. TOPS was founded in 1948 by a Milwaukee housewife, Esther S. Manz. All TOPS members are required to see their physician and get a weight goal from him before beginning classes.

TOPS considers itself akin in spirit to Alcoholics Anonymous, with members keeping in touch between meetings by phone calls, cards, and visits. Programs are sometimes very social in nature, with singing and skits related to weight control. Medical supervision is encouraged during dieting. There are no paid lecturers. Each TOPS group elects a leader from within the group who receives training from supervisors and in workshops. Professionals such as physicians and dietitians are often called on to be program speakers.

"It's like being an alcoholic—you can't cure it [that craving for food]. You can control it." Shirley Cohen, a registered nurse from Towson, Maryland, explained her reason for belonging to TOPS. TOPS fees are the lowest of the diet clubs—$7 a year for the first two years and $5 annually thereafter. There are no other fees, but voluntary contributions are encouraged.

Weight Watchers. The largest of the diet clubs, with over a million members, was begun in 1963 by Jean Nidetch, who had been attending an obesity clinic in New York. Weight Watchers has grown through franchises. In order to get a franchise, "You've had to live through the problem," explained Norma Malis, who established the Baltimore franchise after successfully completing the Weight Watchers program. All lecturers are also required to have been through the program, reached their goal weight, and maintained it. Members are weighed in at weekly meetings and then listen to a Weight Watchers lecture. The fee is $3–5 for the first meeting and $2–4 a week thereafter (rates vary according to franchise). Weight Watchers has marketed special low-calorie foods that can be bought in local supermarkets. The club gives out its own diets—one for men, one for women, and one for teen-agers. Also, special recipes.

Many people who did not do well on the Weight Watchers Diet, mainly because they just couldn't stomach the mandatory high number of fish meals and one liver meal each week, did extremely well on my Easy No-Risk Diet because of its variety. At the same time they attended the Weight

Watchers meeting for reinforcement. The meeting acted as the "policeman" they needed.

Diet Workshop. Trying harder as number two, club leaders are encouraged to impart zeal and enthusiasm and to take a personal interest in dieters who come to workshop meetings. Begun by Lois Lindauer in 1966 in Newton, Massachusetts, the Diet Workshop is also an organization of franchises requiring a $5 member's registration fee and $2 per weekly meeting. Classes begin with mild muscle-toning exercises. Class size is limited to seventy-five. Instructors are trained and certified by Diet Workshop and must maintain their own goal weight in order to keep their jobs. Diet Workshop also gives out separate diets for men, women, and teen-agers, along with special menus. Diet Workshop's national research director, Edith Berman, believes in absorbing the whole body in dieting through an occasional week's visit to a health spa. Mrs. Berman organizes these visits for dieters and also conducts small psychology seminars.

Lois Lindauer, now a size 5, says, "I'm still obese. Not because of my weight, but because food is still as important to me as it is to all fatties." She offered these tips for successful dieting in an interview:

- When you're hungry—eat. Just substitute low-calorie snacks that you have prepared ahead of time. This way you never feel deprived—you never feel you're a martyr.
- Chocolate Alba candy. It's so quick, and it's the real antidote for chocolate addicts. Mix 10 teaspoons water, 1½ teaspoons vanilla, and 1 package Alba dry chocolate skimmed milk into a thick paste. Roll into half-inch balls and freeze.
- Fruit 'n chocolate treat. Mix ½ can pineapple in its own juice with 1 envelope chocolate Alba 77. Spread mixture on aluminum foil and freeze it.
- Lois makes two points in urging you to make special

165

low-calorie dessert snacks: First—Not everyone can substitute something sour when they really want something sweet. Second—You can learn to substitute snacks of a like nature and *try new things*. You have to reeducate your eating process. Try combining tuna fish, cottage cheese, and horseradish for lunch.

- If your motivation for eating is a desire to reward yourself—go out and buy a new lipstick or piece of jewelry instead of a hot fudge sundae.

- Try measuring yourself in some vital places. A good incentive is to keep a graph. Watch that line spiraling downward.

- When you're boiling water for tea or coffee in the morning, it takes two minutes extra to stir up some dietetic jello. Put it in the refrigerator so it will be ready for an afternoon snack.

- A hobby that keeps your hands busy—like needlecraft or knitting—is a mainstay when you might otherwise drift to the refrigerator out of boredom, looking for temporary distraction.

- Take your own vial of dietetic herb salad dressing with you in your pocketbook to restaurants. Sprinkle the herbs on and drown them with a shower from a twist of lemon. Otherwise, while you might feel noble eating a tossed salad, you could be ruining your whole meal plan with a couple of tablespoons of regular high-calorie salad dressing.

- *Don't test your willpower. If you had a lot of it you wouldn't need a diet in the first place.*

Many members and employees of diet clubs are convinced obesity is a life-long hazard that cannot be ignored, but *can* be conquered—through daily attention to what they eat. That is why all three clubs have a maintenance plan for members. Reaching your goal weight is one big victory. But maintaining it each day can be your special little victory.

TEN TIPS FROM SUCCESSFUL DIETERS, MANY OF THEM MY PATIENTS

Some may help you, others not, since your individual psychology plays such an important role in dieting.

1. Look in the mirror and concentrate on your really good qualities.

2. Think of someone you love to be with and to have notice you, then tell yourself, "I won't eat this!"

3. Use smaller dishes for yourself than those you give your family at mealtime.

4. When the urge to cheat strikes, take a walk, bicycle ride, or phone a friend. Diverting your attention may make you forget about food.

5. Try on your old clothes that were sizes bigger to remind yourself how far you've come—or try on something that's still too tight for you, but that you'd *love* to be able to wear.

6. Banish all junk foods from the house.

7. Limit between-meal snacks to fruit or vegetables or special low-calorie recipes. Raw vegetables, especially cauliflower, taste better with seasoned salt sprinkled on them. Try Jane's Crazy Mixed-Up Salt.

8. Don't make your child clean his plate. You could be starting a bad habit for him. All those starving children wherever they are won't benefit from *your* child's getting fat.

9. Anyone living alone can get accustomed to snacking instead of eating regular meals—*and pay the price nutritionally.* One good idea is to cook as though you were preparing a large meal for a family. Then eat a regular portion of everything and store the remainder in aluminum trays—the kind TV dinners come in. Put a serving of meat in one section, vegetables in another, and so forth. Then freeze them. And you've done the cooking for three, four, or five nutritionally sound dinners for the future.

10. Don't feel you have to make up excuses to hide the fact that you're dieting. Take your own diet soda with you to parties, even wedding receptions, to avoid drinking alcohol. You have the right to try to be your healthiest and best-looking and happiest. Be true to yourself.

UNDERSTANDING YOURSELF

How well do you really know yourself? When you're alone do you always have either the radio, stereo, or television set going? Take some time to contemplate. Knowing yourself and understanding what motivates you to overeat are essential in order to learn how to curb the tendencies. Here are nine cases of specific problems that were solved when some dieters kept the diary, recommended in Chapter 6, to find out what the problem was:

Eat Sweets at Time of Crisis?

Paul, a boyish twenty-seven-year-old airline pilot from Chattanooga, was referred to me by the company physician. His problem was that he would eat sweets under stress. Even in the cockpit of his airplane, he kept a box of chocolates beside him to satisfy his mouth and soothe his nerves when he ran into problems. (Of course, better that he ate the chocolate than let the crisis affect his thinking while piloting the airplane.)

Solution to the problem: Instead of eating the chocolates I had Paul use a sugar substitute. He put it on his tongue. Sometimes nothing more than a little bit of saccharine on the tip of his tongue would take away his insatiable desire for sweets.

Eat Late at Night?

James, a leather tanner from Albany, New York, always did well until late at night. He would get up at night and walk around while others in the family slept. The only thing that seemed to satisfy him was to raid the refrigerator.

The solution: Whenever he opened the refrigerator door, James would always find foods that appealed to him. So I had him put those tempting foods in opaque containers and at the *back* of the refrigerator so he couldn't see them. He wrapped cellophane around the foods he was *allowed* to eat as snacks, such as cubes of cold meat that had been left over from the day before, or pieces of chicken and fish, and vegetables. And they went up front and center in the refrigerator.

Snack too Much?

William, thirty-eight, a commercial painter with a prematurely salt-and-pepper crew cut, was referred to me from Dallas by his local doctor. William's problem was that he grabbed a quick snack every day for a fast pickup.

His solution: Substituting diet cola for the snack. He still got his pickup, but with fewer calories. (Pour your diet soda over cracked ice and eat the ice too).

Do Bread and Dessert Do You In?

John, a forty-one-year-old insurance agent from New Orleans, had no problem staying on his diet as long as his wife prepared the proper food for him. But his job took him away from home often and he ate out quite a bit in restaurants. He developed a real fondness for the sourdough bread, butter, rolls, and crock of cheese served before the meal, and the desserts beckoning from the ever-lit glass case.

Solution to the problem: He asked the waiter not to bring anything to the table except the main meal—and with it, the check. So dessert was no longer feasible.

Are You an All-Day Nibbler?

Laura, thirty-three, a housewife with three children from Hartford, found her problem was that while she cleaned the table at the end of a meal, she nibbled on the leftover food. She just couldn't stand to see it go to waste. Solving her problem was simple. She now gets her children to clear the table and any nibbling is done by them. Since they are all underweight, it has worked out fine.

Get Hungry Before Dinner?

Tom, thirty-six, from Hialeah, worked at the racetrack, and always beat his wife home from work by two hours. He had twenty-seven extra pounds on his 6 foot 1 inch medium frame. Tom's problem was raiding the refrigerator while waiting for his wife to arrive and fix dinner. So he decided on certain days of the week he would work out in the gym for the two hours before his wife got home from work.

Overeat at Parties?

A minister from Austin attended a lot of receptions and social functions and said he felt awkward if he didn't eat all the food offered him. He didn't want to offend anyone. But his weight had pushed up thirty-nine pounds over his ideal 160 pounds. So he decided to put very little food on his plate at these receptions and to spread it over a very large surface. That way he satisfied his hostesses while stabilizing his weight.

Do You Like Your Own Cooking Too Much?

Mary sells handbags in Minneapolis. Large boned and 5 feet 6 inches tall, she should have weighed 149, but was twenty pounds overweight. She had an obsession for trying new recipes. And when she did, she simply overate them. She could not bear to waste anything she had made. Now, when the urge is just too strong, she offers to make a meal for a friend and freezes the leftovers.

Do You Buy the Wrong Food?

A thirty-three-year-old bachelor who lived alone and assisted with the Watergate investigation, had had it with fat, and decided to find out what he was doing wrong. He weighed 263 instead of the 202 pounds his large, 6 foot 4 inch frame could best handle. He often went shopping in the Washington supermarkets on impulse when he was hungry and bought a lot of junk foods from the well-stocked shelves. He couldn't wait to get home and consume his booty. Solution: He now makes a list of exactly what he needs in advance and he *only* buys those specific foods. He also never goes out to shop except on a full stomach.

QUESTIONS COMMONLY ASKED

● *Exactly what are empty calories?*

This is a term that describes the calories in foods without any other nutritional value. In other words these foods contain no vitamins or minerals, just calories without nutrition. That is why the calories are referred to as empty. Soda pop is a good example. It is something that all dieters should ruthlessly cut out.

- *Should you eat margarine instead of butter?*

From a calorie standpoint, believe it or not, there are just as many calories in margarine as there are in butter. But *less saturated fat* in margarine than in butter. So, if you have a tendency toward a heart condition, it is better to use soft margarine, particularly one high in polyunsaturated fatty acids such as Fleischmann's corn oil margarine or Promise.

- *Does exercise help you lost weight?*

The answer is emphatically yes. But don't look to massive weight loss from exercise, because it takes a *lot* of exercise to melt away the fat. It is true that exercise will burn up some calories. The main and vitally important thing exercise does, though, is make you feel better, help you with better posture, and a better-looking body.

- *How can you avoid getting flabby as you lose weight?*

The only answer to this *is* exercise—especially focusing on those parts of the body which are the flabbiest. In addition, good posture will hide a lot of flabbiness. By dieting gradually, losing about two pounds a week, your skin will condition itself to the loss of fat it covers. It cannot adapt quickly enough, however, if you lose a lot of pounds fast on a crash diet.

- *What do you do if you get constipated on a diet?*

You may have fewer bowel movements because you are eating less, but this is not constipation. Constipation means that in the bowel movements you do have, the stool itself is very hard and the bowel movement sometimes painful. If this is true, then increase your water intake and eat more raw vegetables for adequate bulk. If this is not sufficient, add a little (between 1 and 2 tablespoons) of unprocessed bran to your daily diet.

• *Is there cause for alarm if a gross change in the menstrual period is experienced when dieting is started?*

That depends on what is being done in addition to dieting. Actually, a change is not unusual. No one really knows the answer, except that most diets do alter the endocrine balance for a while. If it is a well-balanced diet, as weight is lost, the periods should return to normal. If they don't after three months, then there may be some gynecological reason, and a doctor should be consulted.

• *How much water should you drink when you are on a diet?*

If you are healthy, you can drink as much water as you wish. You will not have a fluid-retention problem from drinking water, if at the same time you don't take in an excessive amount of salt. Remember, the more water you drink, the more you will eliminate, providing you have normal kidneys and a normal heart. Be sure to drink a glass of water before each meal.

• *Do adults need to drink milk?*

Although it is true your bones are formed when you reach adulthood, it is also true that you are constantly losing and replacing calcium from your bones. You need this calcium, and milk is a perfectly good source. I would suggest you have two glasses of milk daily or use two dairy shares. The only contraindication to this would be if you develop diarrhea soon after drinking milk, you may lack an enzyme needed to digest milk. If your doctor says this is the case, ask him for a substitute. There are adequate calcium substitutes currently available. A high percentage of certain races and nationalities, usually dark-complexioned races, do lack this enzyme. If you think you fall into either of these categories, be sure you have your doctor's advice on any diet.

Milk can supply all the essential requirements for the human body except iron and vitamin C. I would suggest you restrict your milk to skimmed rather than whole milk. This will significantly decrease the fat in it as well as the calories. Reconstituted powdered skimmed milk is the lowest in fat. It takes about ten days to get used to its taste. But once you are, you really don't have any desire for regular milk.

● *Does fish have more protein than meat per unit weight?*

There is about ½ ounce more protein in a pound of flatfish, such as flounder or sole, than in a pound of choice beef (that is, beef without the bone). But a pound of beef gives you 1,400 calories and a pound of fish gives you less than 350 calories. So if there is a choice, a pound of fish will give you more protein and far less calories.

● *Is it okay to skip a meal?*

No. Many people who do skip have the tendency either to nibble later on or overeat at the next meal and actually end up consuming more calories for the day. Skipping a meal can also cause a headache, irritability, and weakness.

● *But there's often no time for breakfast. Isn't it all right to skip that?*

My answer to this is a flat no—simply because of the twenty-five people that I studied at Johns Hopkins who skipped breakfast. They *all* ate more calories during that day for the simple reason that when people ignore breakfast, they build up what I call "hidden hunger" that increases as the day progresses and they end up consuming more calories than if they had eaten a good breakfast. *Breakfast is the most important meal of the day* because your body has been without food for its longest period and needs refueling.

● *To follow the Easy, No-Risk Diet I need to know what represents 3 ounces of meat or whatever proportion of meat is called for. Is there some simple way I can determine this?*

Yes. You can purchase a small, inexpensive scale, like a postage scale, and measure your food on it. It is perfectly accurate.

● *Is there any way I can get an idea of portion size—even roughly—other than by weighing my meat?*

Yes. There are 16 ounces to a pound. *Raw* meat, fish, or poultry lose weight when they are cooked. Copy this table to hang in your kitchen.

3 ounces cooked meat or 3 protein shares is equal to:

4 ounces raw meat—no bone
4 ounces raw fish—no bone

5 ounces each lamb, veal, pork chops
(cut 3 per pound in order to get
3 ounces cooked weight)

½ large chicken breast—cooked
1 chicken thigh plus 1 drumstick—cooked

¾ cup boneless, cooked, flaked, chopped meat, poultry
or fish

4 X 3 X ½ inches slice of cooked roast beef, veal, lamb,
pork, or ham

• *If I drink more than three cups of coffee a day I get very nervous. Should I limit the amount of coffee or tea I drink daily?*

It is true that coffee and tea contain considerable caffeine. Caffeine may cause nervousness, sweating, irritability, fast heartbeat, and stomachaches. You may wish to limit your intake after consulting with your doctor.

• *What is the caffeine content of some common beverages?*

The following beverages contain caffeine. Be sure to read the labels. Though beware, if you are a caffeine-sensitive person. Not all colas list it. So familiarize yourself with the following:

mg of caffeine in 1 fluid ounce

Coca-Cola	4.00
Diet Pepsi	3.00
Diet Rite Cola	3.50
Dr. Pepper	5.30
Pepsi-Cola	3.00
Royal Crown Cola	3.50
Tab	4.00

By comparison:

Coffee	10.16
Tea	12.00
Decaf (Nestle)	0.03
Nescafe (Nestle)	1.17
Sanka	0.55

Multiply the above figures by how many ounces you are drinking so that you can see how much caffeine you are taking in.

● *I drink a lot of cola to fill me up so I won't eat so much food during the meal. Is this a good idea?*

No. Because colas contain sugar and have too many calories. A 12-ounce bottle of regular cola contains about 145 calories. Ginger ale has only about 115 calories. Even most diet colas contain some sugar, although very little—read the label to see how many calories you are getting. If you are going to drink soft drinks, choose a diet soda that does not exceed 5 calories in each bottle or can. Read the label. *Club soda has no calories.* Beef or chicken bouillon dissolved in hot water makes a satisfying between-meal snack and is relatively calorie-free.

● *Would it be better for me to drink fruit juice than cola?*

Yes. Fresh orange juice contains 110 calories per cup. Fruit juices contain vitamins, minerals, and calories. Canned orange juice, sweetened, has 135 calories. Grape juice has 240 calories per cup. Fresh or canned unsweetened grapefruit juice has only 80 calories a cup. If it is sweetened, it contains 130 calories a cup. Tomato juice has only 50 calories per cup. Therefore, if you like juices, I would suggest tomato juice. It is also rich in vitamin C. Count fruit juices including tomato as a fruit share. Have you thought, though, about quenching your thirst with water? Remember, you should drink 4 glasses of water a day.

● *I like lemon. Is this high in calories?*

It is better than drinking cola. A whole cup of pure lemon juice contains 60 calories. You can dilute one part of pure lemon juice with four parts of water or soda, add some sugar substitute, and have a nice refreshing drink. The juice of one lemon contains 49 calories. But if you take that juice and add sugar to it to make lemonade, you add about 50 calories for every tablespoon of sugar. If you use a frozen concentrate with sugar to make lemonade, you are drinking 885 calories per can.

● *I was told there are less calories in Irish whisky than in gin. Is this so?*

No. There is virtually no difference in calories between gin, rum, scotch, and Irish whisky. A shot glass of 1½ ounces of almost any 86-proof liquor contains about 110 calories.

● *I recently abandoned grasshoppers for brandy Alexanders because I was told they contain less calories. Is this true?*

Unfortunately not. Brandy Alexanders, grasshoppers, or other fancy drinks containing sugar plus cream zoom up to about 300 calories per drink. Sweet liqueurs all by themselves contain about 100 calories per ounce. Martinis have 140 calories. Manhattans 165 calories. A Tom Collins or a whisky sour contains 225 calories. So alcoholic drinks are loaded with calories.

● *What is something good to mix with my alcoholic drink if I don't want to add calories?*

The best thing is water, or try club soda with or without a sugar substitute. Quinine water adds 88 calories for an 8-ounce glass. Bitter lemon or bitter orange adds 125 calories for each 8-ounce glass. Your portion of wine plus soda makes a pleasing combination.

● *What is a good nonalcoholic drink that doesn't have too many calories?*

Water is the best. Iced tea with lemon is good. Iced coffee, either black or with a twist of lemon, is tasty and low in calories. Teas flavored with orange and spices, such as Constant Comment taste good hot or cold. Or you can order an LS or an LW—that is, a lime with soda or lime with water, with or without sugar substitute.

● *How important is iodine in my diet?*

In order to burn calories normally you must have iodine in your diet. This prevents goiter, which is a lump in the neck due to a malfunctioning, enlarged thyroid gland. Use iodized salt unless your doctor tells you that you are allergic to iodine. Eating shellfish will also supply iodine. If you live in the states of Washington, Oregon, Montana, Idaho, Utah, Wyoming, Wisconsin, or Michigan, be aware that there is a lack of iodine in the soil. This is also true of certain areas in Colorado, North Dakota, Minnesota, Iowa, Illinois, Indiana, Ohio, and West Virginia. By using iodized salt instead of plain salt in your cooking, you can fulfill your iodine needs.

● *I have a problem handling salt near my menstrual period. I get bloated. My doctor told me to keep my salt intake down. What foods should I avoid?*

You should be seeing your doctor for a precise regimen tailored to your needs. Remember, salt is sodium chloride. For a minor temporary problem, you should avoid foods that are preserved or processed with sodium chloride or any

179

chemical that contains sodium. Because of the number of people requiring a sodium restriction, the manufacturers must list the sodium content. *Read labels carefully.* You should avoid the following foods that have a high salt content: anchovies, bacon and bacon fat, chipped or corned beef, regular bouillon cubes, celery salt, canned soups, all cheeses, dried cod, frankfurters, ham, herring, meat extracts, meat sauces, meat tenderizers, luncheon meats, prepared mustard, olives, pickles, salted popcorn, potato chips, pretzels, relishes, salt at the table, salt in smoked meats, salt in smoked fish, garlic salt, onion salt, sardines, sausages, soy sauce. Also, use a light hand when cooking with salt and use salt that is iodized.

8

PLATEAU—

WHAT TO DO

WHEN STALLED

Reaching a plateau is fine if you're rock climbing.

But the plateau is the dread of every dieter. It's that point where some dieters level off and quit losing temporarily.

Some people are lucky and just keep losing until they reach their ideal weight. Others lose from plateau to plateau. In other words, they may remain at a plateau temporarily and then suddenly lose some more. They become accustomed to losing weight in this fashion and to them the plateau is no real cause for alarm; however, many less-fortunate dieters hit a plateau, and their weight just doesn't budge. It is *this* dieter with whom we are mainly concerned.

First of all we assume you are still strongly motivated and ask that you check on yourself honestly. Have you become "tired" of your diet and gradually drifted off it? Do you look so much better at your lower weight that you are subconsciously rewarding yourself with a little something extra? Where is your diet diary? Can you find it?

Many chronic "plateauers" are really lax. They trust to memory for too much, and memory can become badly faded, especially about something as basically unpleasant as a diet. In any case, dig out the basic diet again and start dieting as you did in the beginning. Keep your shares lists in front of you to make sure you are really following them correctly.

Get out your measuring cups and scales and start using *them* again. Approximate portions are no good at this time. Really measure out that ½ cup or weigh those 4 ounces. Many dieters' approximations grow in a direct ratio to the length of time since the last measurements were made.

Sylvia, a sixty-year-old manufacturing company employee from Evanston, Indiana, weighed 115 pounds. Her 5 foot 2 inch, small frame could only carry 106 pounds well and at that weight she was very attractive with her short, frosted hair. She went on the Easy, No-Risk Diet and in the first month lost five pounds, dropping to 110 pounds. Then she hit a plateau and for the next two weeks did not lose any weight. Sylvia couldn't understand why, since she really *thought* she was following the same regimen she had previously followed.

True with one crucial exception: Rather than measuring cupfuls or half cups, Sylvia would estimate—better, "guesstimate"—pouring from various boxes. When she went back and started measuring what she had been guesstimating, she found she was off by a good 20 percent. In other words, she was pouring and eating 20 percent more than she should have been. That amount accounted for the increased number of hidden calories that prevented her from losing weight. As soon as she went back to her accurate measuring, Sylvia started losing once again, and in six weeks she was down to her ideal weight of 106 pounds.

Q. You can get really disgusted if you weigh every morning and the scale doesn't move. How often should you weigh, and what should you do if you don't lose?

A. Give yourself a week on your renewed regimen and *then* weigh yourself. If you haven't lost, there may be another problem. This, many times, is hidden salt. If an increased amount of salt is present in your diet, the cells which have lost fat will partially fill with water and your weight loss will stop. Also, one of the byproducts of fat breakdown is water, and this water too will fill up empty cells in the presence of excess salt. The obvious solution to this problem is to cut down on the salt in your diet.

We have found that if you go on salt-free liquids for twenty-four hours, much of the excess salt, along with the surplus fluid, will leave your system. *But, before doing this, make sure you get your doctor's permission.* Try using only water, coffee and tea, along with special *salt-free* bouillon, diet soda and salt-free diet jello. After the twenty-four hours, return to the Easy, No-Risk Diet and eliminate *all* salt, even in cooking, for three days. This would, of course, include all Accent, monosodium glutamate, Seasonal, soy sauce, and foods high in salt content such as sausage, frankfurter, cheese, luncheon meats, Chinese food, etc. Even just a tiny "taste" of these high-salt foods can be disastrous. *You may not count it, but nature does.* Bear in mind, too, that all restaurant food is prepared with both salt and butter, which may itself be high in salt. Once you are losing again, cook lightly with salt, more highly with spices and herbs, and do not add salt at the table. This regimen should, of course, first be approved by your doctor, whom you should see if you have stayed on the low-salt diet and have *not* lost weight. You may have some sort of metabolic imbalance that requires his help.

Q. How can you tell if a food is very high in salt?

A. A good rule to remember is that a food that tastes excessively salty most likely is excessively salty.

Marguerite, a thirty-six-year-old fur goods saleslady from Hammond, Indiana, is 5 feet 6 inches tall and weighs 140 pounds. She burned 2,176 calories a day. The weight she felt best at for her medium frame was 125 pounds. So she went on the Easy, No-Risk Diet, and after two weeks of easy dieting, dropped to 134 pounds. Then she hit a plateau and for the next ten days did not lose an ounce. She couldn't understand why until, thoroughly studying her diary, she found that the only major substitution was that she was now using more bouillon cubes. Regular bouillon cubes contain salt. It was that hidden salt that was causing her to retain fluids and show no apparent weight loss. She went off the bouillon cubes, substituting salt-free bouillon in their stead and once again started losing weight. Now two months later she has reached her ideal weight of 125 pounds—looks and feels great.

The main thing to bear in mind is not to give up. When you hit a plateau, diet more strenuously and become even more determined. Your doctor will be glad to help you over the rough periods, as long as you are honest both with him and yourself. Honesty and determination nearly always conquer the plateau.

Q. Is it true that as you lose weight you burn up less calories, and therefore make additional weight loss more difficult?

A. Yes. Because the amount of weight you lose is equal to the number of calories you burn up in excess of the number of calories you eat. The more weight you lose, the less calories your body burns up. Therefore, as you lose weight you should exercise more. For the more you exercise, the more calories you will burn and the more weight you will lose.

John, a twenty-seven-year-old Camden, New Jersey, electric equipment manufacturer, had a large frame, and his ideal weight was determined to be 170 pounds. He weighed 250 pounds and burned a whopping 4,020 calories a day. He went on our basic diet and at the end of the first month, still staying on the diet, he weighed 220 pounds. At the end of the second month, still on the diet, he weighed 200 pounds —looked better and felt better. At the end of the third month he weighed 192 pounds.

But now he became depressed because he had lost only 8 pounds during the third month. Yet he swore he stayed on the diet religiously and, indeed, this was true. The reason he lost so much during the first month was that he had experienced a great excess fluid loss along with the fat loss. The second month he still had some fluid loss, but by the time the third month rolled around he was carrying less weight and therefore burning less calories. He also had no additional excess fluid to lose. Since the number of calories you burn decreases as you lose weight, he was burning up more calories when he weighed 250 pounds than when he weighed 192 pounds. Therefore, staying on the same diet and everything else being equal, he would lose less weight when he weighed 192 pounds. When I explained this to John, he realized what the problem was . . . that in fact there really *was* no problem. He was losing at just the rate he should. He kept losing, and after three additional months he has reached his ideal weight of 170 pounds. At this weight and on the Figure-Keeper maintenance regimen he is doing very well.

Q. Can constipation be a factor in plateau?
A. Yes. It can also make you feel sluggish, less determined, and give you headaches.

Joseph, a 6 foot 1 inch knitting-mill worker from Atlanta, does his best work at 170 pounds but had reached 185 pounds, and for that reason went on our basic diet. At the end of the first month he weighed 175 pounds and felt fine.

Then he hit a plateau and stayed there. An analysis of what he was eating showed he wasn't cheating on his diet. But Joe did notice one thing. He had become severely constipated. For this reason his doctor added one teaspoon a day of unprocessed bran to his diet. During the first week Joe had some flatulence and a bit of discomfort, but this was over by the second week. He felt well and had normal bowel movements. Within one month, continuing to have normal bowel movements, he reached his ideal weight of 170 pounds and has stayed there since.

Dr. Hugh Trowell, reporting in the *American Journal of Clinical Nutrition,* believes that fibers not only can help you become more regular, but can also prevent such ailments as cancer of the colon, appendicitis, colitis, and diverticular disease. I could find no objective substantiation of this claim, although many physicians do believe in their patients using unprocessed bran. (An interesting side note is that many people who get constipated using "grass" get unconstipated using unprocessed bran.)

Q. How important is measuring food portions?

A. Marguerite, thirty-three, employee from a newspaper in Bridgeport, Connecticut, reached a plateau. A careful history of the way she prepared food was very revealing. She would sift flour into a large glass bowl and then pack it down. She would then transfer *heaping* teaspoons when the recipe merely called for teaspoons.

In measuring you should always sift flour onto aluminum foil or a piece of waxed paper and then spoon or scoop it lightly into a marked measuring cup. Do not pack it down. Also, you should always use level, not heaping teaspoonfuls.

Marguerite's history further revealed that when a recipe called for milk or other liquid ingredients she would measure them looking *down* at the cup. This is not the correct way to do it. You should measure all liquid ingredients at eye level. Just analyzing what she'd been doing, and also realizing that she didn't have a true appreciation of some common interconversions of weights and measures, was a big help to Marguerite. Once she paid attention to these details she started losing again and has continued to lose.

Common information it is essential to know:

> 1 tablespoon = 3 teaspoons
> 2 tablespoons = 1 ounce or 1 jigger or 30 cc (cubic centimeters)
> 4 tablespoons = ¼ cup
> 8 tablespoons = ½ cup
> 16 tablespoons = 1 cup
> 1 cup = ½ pint or ½ pound
> 2 cups = 1 pint or 1 pound
> 2 pints = 1 quart or 2 pounds
> 4 quarts = 1 gallon or 8 pounds
> 16 ounces = 1 pound
> 16 fluid ounces = 1 pint or 2 cups

It is important to post this information near your refrigerator or near your cupboard—somewhere in the kitchen where you can have ready reference to it when you are measuring your food portions.

Unless you have a medical problem, following our simple advice about *really* staying on your diet and paying careful attention to accurate food measurement will allow you to move off the plateau and start losing weight once again.

9

IN MY

CONSULTING ROOM—

MEDICAL PROBLEMS

AND OVERWEIGHT

No diet ever works for you? You've gone here, there, and everywhere? You lost some weight. You gained it back. You're disgusted. There seem to be no definite answers for you. Now, you have tried my basic diet, my version of the basic diet for carboholics, even my minidiet. You read, understood, and followed my tips for losing weight and nothing seems to really work. Then we have to face the facts. *You may have a metabolic or endocrine disorder that directly interferes with your ability to lose weight.*

The only way you are going to be helped is to find a competent specialist willing to take the time to get to the bottom of your particular problem. He could be your local doctor, an internist (a doctor who specializes in the practice of internal medicine), an endocrinologist (a doctor who specializes in glands that affect your metabolism) or a well-trained and dedicated bariatrician (a doctor who limits practice to treatment of obesity). Call your local medical society and ask if any doctors in your area are doing work on obesity. In the next few pages I will share with you things I look for in my private practice. Armed with this knowledge, you will know how to find a specialist who really leaves no stone unturned in discovering your problem and correcting or arresting it.

My approach is not unique. It is the approach of any good endocrinologist. The first thing I do when you come to see me is sit down with you and listen and talk to you. This results in the compilation of a 14-page history. It is immensely important for me to know everything I can of medical significance about you, from the time you were conceived until the present—starting with the state of your mother's health during her pregnancy and whether you were a large or small baby, because babies born over nine pounds are suspected of having diabetes mellitus (sugar diabetes).

Not only should *you* be checked, but your parents should also be checked for diabetes shortly after delivery. Large babies are suspected of not handling carbohydrates properly, as are their parents. This does not mean this will be the case, but it alerts my index of suspicion so that the necessary tests are done. If you and your parents were not checked at your birth, it is not too late for all of you to be checked now. It is also important to know if you were breast or bottle fed and whether you were fat as a child.

From a careful history I can get an idea as to whether you were born with an increased number of fat cells or you became fat later in life. This is important in order to project the prognosis of the obesity and to help me in counseling you. If you were not fat as a child, did you become fat at puberty? Did emotional problems cause you to overeat? Did you suddenly start to gain an inordinate amount of weight after some physical or emotional trauma? Did you gain excessively after a surgical procedure, such as a tonsilectomy? What was your weight when you married? What was your weight five years later? What is it now? What has happened to you during your adult life? Have you gradually gained weight during middle age? If you're a woman, have you gained it mostly in your thighs and hips? Do you have an increased amount of hair on your face and if so when did you first notice it? Do you have an abnormal distribution of hair on your body, particularly around your nipples? Do you have acne? Are your periods regular and normal? If you're a man, have you put pounds on mainly around your beltline?

Do you have an abnormal distribution of fat, such as a hump in the back of your neck? Do you have thin arms and legs but a heavy body? Or are you light from the waist up and heavy from the waist down?

Are you excessively tired or excessively weak? Do you become irritable or tired after you eat certain foods, especially carbohydrates? Do you perspire a lot? Does your heart race? Have you had trouble in the past with nails being brittle and cracking? Has your skin been excessively dry and sometimes rough? Has your hair been falling out excessively, recently? Do you have a dry scalp? Did you find yourself terribly cold, even before the energy crisis? At night, do you find yourself wanting more covers than your mate? Do you prefer the warmer summertime over the wintertime because you are cold? These are but a few sample questions I ask. The whole idea is to know you and your problems.

Taking a good history made diagnosis possible of Freddie, a thirty-one-year-old mailman from Albany, New York. He never had a weight problem until his wife told him she had found a twenty-two-year-old hippie and was going to run away with him. Then Fred began to overeat. Over the next six months he gained fifty-seven pounds. He would buy large amounts of candy, especially licorice, in a confectionery store, and then eat it as he delivered his mail. He noticed that over the past three months he had become very forgetful and that his legs were growing weaker and weaker and starting to become painful. It became so bad that he actually found himself dragging his feet. Finally he had to take sick leave because he couldn't continue with his work. When I saw him, he walked with a shuffling gait, had difficulty elevating his legs, and underactive reflexes. His blood showed he had a deficiency of potassium, which I found was due to his eating an inordinate amount of licorice. The licorice caused him to lose his potassium through urination.

Put on the Easy, No-Risk Diet, and taken off the licorice, he did very well. His potassium returned quickly to normal and in 5½ months he became less forgetful and returned to his ideal weight. It is true his wife has left him, but Fred has now found a new life with another woman and as soon as his divorce is complete he plans to marry her. The clue to his diagnosis was that he ate an inordinate amount of licorice, which is known to cause potassium depletion and subsequently reversible muscle problems.

A more common cause of forgetfulness in the overweight person is hypothyroidism. Four percent of fat people have low thyroid function. Doris is a thirty-one-year-old schoolteacher from Houston. She always enjoyed teaching until two years ago when she became very forgetful—mainly forgetting assignments from one day to the next. She also tired easily and started missing school two and three days a month. She could hardly wait until the end of the school day so she could go home and to bed. She also noticed she was becoming much less interested in sex. In fact, sex really didn't much matter to her anymore. Her husband told her she was developing fat deposits above her collarbone, around her waist, and at her ankles. Previously she never had trouble with skin infections, but she now noticed that she would often develop what she called boils. For the first time in her life she was troubled by swelling of her fingers, breasts, and the area around her ankles. When I saw her she was about fifteen pounds overweight. Her skin was dry, her tongue thick. Appropriate tests showed she did have hypothyroidism and was deficient in thyroid hormone. Put on thyroid hormone in the exact amount she needed and on an appropriate diet, Doris has done well, losing about fifteen pounds in two months, and keeping it off now for two and a half years.

After the history is completed, I do a thorough physical examination except for a pelvic. I start at the top of the head and finish at the bottom of the toes. It was the findings from a thorough physical examination on Betty that led to her correct diagnosis. She is a former twenty-two-year-old Disney World employee from Anaheim, California, with short dark brown hair and brown eyes. She was sixty-four pounds overweight. Betty had an aggressive personality, probably compensation for her ungainly physical appearance. She had a round, full face with an excess amount of facial hair and an excess of hair on her arms and legs. She had acne on her face and talked huskily. She had been married for three years and desperately wanted to become pregnant. Her menstrual periods were very irregular, and over the last year she noted that she had developed an unusual amount of facial hair, as well as some hair between her breasts and under her navel. Her acne came and went but was far worse during the last six months, when she also noticed pain on both sides of her lower abdomen. On physical examination, her blood pressure was elevated (170/100) and a careful pelvic examination suggested that both her ovaries were enlarged.

I diagnosed Betty as having the Stein-Leventhal Syndrome. She had all its characteristics—she was obese, had excessive body hair, high blood pressure, was infertile, had irregular menstrual periods, and multiple ovarian cysts. Chemical testing also showed she had a lack of a female hormone and too much male hormone. After consultation with a surgeon, it was decided that the best procedure was surgical reduction of the size of her ovaries. This was accomplished, and two years postoperatively and after dieting, Betty has achieved her ideal weight.

For the first time during her adult life she saw results from dieting. There was a complete reversal of her symptoms. Although the excess hair on her face did not go away, she did not grow any additional hair, and after ultra-high frequency treatment for its removal, the facial hair has not returned. But most importantly, she became pregnant and has delivered a normal six-pound baby girl.

After completion of the physical examination, I then analyze a strand of your hair. I can tell a great deal from just looking at the hair. It can give me clues to possible vitamin or mineral deficiencies. I can test for the strength of the hair, and examine the hair root under the microscope. This gives me a clue to your protein status and the blood supply to your scalp. Just as during the physical examination, by looking into your eyes, I can find clues to many diseases, from leukemia to diabetes, so I can get many clues by looking at your hair.

For example, if you have a protein deficiency, you might have hair that shows less color, and your hair roots might be decreased in size and strength.

I then do an oxygen consumption test (explained in Chapter 1). This helped determine what was wrong with Sharon, a lovely redhead with hazel eyes from Boston. She is a twenty-one-year-old graduate student in psychology. Over the past two years she had gained thirty-seven pounds. She noticed increased fatigue, decreased mobility, and she felt increased sensitivity to cold. She had started sleeping with her electric blanket turned up high. She had noticed that her fingernails split and were quite brittle, and she had dry scalp and skin. Her periods, for no apparent reason, became irregular. She went to the school doctor who, because of the above symptoms and the thirty-seven-pound weight gain, thought she had low thyroid. He did a conventional PBI (protein bound iodine) blood test for thyroid and found it was normal.

I repeated the tests and did indeed find that Sharon's PBI registered normal, but her oxygen consumption test showed she was only burning 945 calories a day. That meant that if she ate more than a measly 945 calories a day, Sharon gained weight. I then knew there had to be something medically wrong. So I renewed my testing procedures and did a T3 (tri-iodothyronine blood test for thyroid). It was low. She was actually suffering from a low T3 which was the cause of her not burning enough calories. Sharon was placed on proper thyroid replacement medication, and was on a diet. On this regimen she lost her thirty-seven pounds in five months and has kept it off now for two and a half years, without the symptoms she previously experienced.

Clues from your history, physical examination, hair analysis, and an oxygen consumption test can lead me to order the necessary other tests, such as blood and urine analysis to find out if you have a specific medical problem causing your obesity. To thoroughly check out your endocrine glands, I will also do a twenty-four-hour urine test, analyzing all the urine you made in that time period. Then, armed with all this information, I can determine whether you have any problems with your endocrine glands—pituitary,

194

thyroid, parathyroid, adrenal, pancreas, or gonads.

When Ruth Powers was forty-eight, her magazine employer suggested she retire to save what health she had. Her doctor gave her a year to live. She weighed 223 pounds and was in a turmoil when she came to see me in November, 1972.

Fourteen months later, an enthusiastic, effervescent Ruth who had dropped from a size 24½ to a 16½ dress, recalled her earlier self: "The only time I lost weight was when I was pregnant," she said. "I went to Weight Watchers four different times and never lost more than eighteen pounds in seven to eight months. I cried myself to sleep every night."

I discovered that Ruth was a diabetic, and gave her proper oral medication and a special diet. Now, while dieting is still hard at times, she is managing it.

A number of other patients were found to have thyroid malfunctions which nurtured their weight problem. On proper medication and diet, they find for the first time that they are significantly losing pounds.

An example of the value of the laboratory tests is the case of Susan, a twenty-nine-year-old blond, blue-eyed housewife from Atlanta. Susan went to her physician because she was thirty-six pounds overweight and had just gone on a high-protein, drink-all-the-alcohol-you-want diet. She lost only three pounds during the first month on the diet, but developed the most unusual array of problems. She became very tired, which she seldom had been before, mentally fatigued (she just felt mentally "wacked out"), irritated (she would start to scream and yell at her husband, which she had rarely done before), and found herself unable to cope with daily problems. It was too much of an effort for her to manage such simple tasks as grocery shopping, taking the car in for repairs, or picking up the children at school. Sometimes she felt profoundly depressed, sometimes anxious. She would wake up in the middle of the night with muscle cramps that would last three to five minutes, and often had palpitations or fast-fluttering heartbeats. She told her doctor about these symptoms. He thought she had an emotional problem and referred her to a psychiatrist for emotional help, and to me to lose thirty-six pounds. Thorough examination including a blood magnesium level revealed she was actually suffering from a magnesium deficiency.

This was the cause both of her emotional and physical problems. In fact, she was a prime candidate for it because of her diet—a high-protein diet and a lot of alcohol. The more protein food you eat, and the more alcohol you drink, the more magnesium you need.

Susan was treated with magnesium, put on my diet, and after four months she lost thirty-six pounds. She now goes out of her way to eat foods high in magnesium although she really needn't, because she gets plenty of magnesium in our Basic Figure-Keeper maintenance diet. The foods that she likes which are rich in magnesium include almonds and other nuts, different types of seeds, such as sunflower, sesame, caraway, and pumpkin, wheat germ, oatmeal, corn meal, and peanut butter.

Lonnie, a thirty-one-year-old barmaid, never had a weight problem until she became pregnant. She gained fifty-two pounds in six months after delivering her first baby. She became tired and forgetful. She went to her physician, who worked her up, but could find nothing wrong with her thyroid and referred her to me for consultation and evaluation. After a thorough examination and analysis of her blood, she was found to have thyroid antibodies and clinical evidence of hypothyroidism. No other test would have revealed this. We treated Lonnie with proper medication, Cytomel. On this regimen and, staying on my basic diet, she has done extremely well. After eight months she lost her fifty-two pounds and has now kept it off for an additional four months.

I also do a test to determine the electrical activity of the heart. This is terribly important because many fat people are prone to heart attacks and sudden death. Ginger, a forty-three-year-old Chicago schoolteacher with short blond hair, brown eyes, round, pudgy face and vibrant smile, thought she was having a heart attack. She would experience hot flashes, sweats, throbbing pains in her head and chest, and a feeling of anxiety. But an electrocardiogram (EKG) and blood tests confirmed my clinical assessment that Ginger showed no apparent evidence of heart problems.

Reassured by the perfectly normal EKG, she then started talking about her children—two boys, ten and thirteen, and one daughter, fifteen. Her ten-year-old son is hyperactive and has a specific learning disability. She spends a great deal of time with him. Last month, out of the blue, her husband told her he no longer loved her and asked for a divorce.

She had just, within the last six months, started menopause and during that time gained twenty-two pounds. Her periods used to be very regular up to a year ago, when they became erratic. Her other menopausal symptoms were then capped by her periods ceasing completely. She experienced four to five hot flashes a day associated with sweats, and had a throbbing, pounding headache at the top of her head most of the time. She also felt an increased pressure on the inside of her head.

During the past four months she gained twenty-two pounds and for the first time had a weight problem. Ginger gained most of the weight in her thighs and around her abdomen. A thorough evaluation showed she was within limits, except for a decreased amount of female hormones as a result of going through menopause. An analysis showed what female hormones she was deficient in, and to what degree. She was placed on the proper female hormones, put on my basic diet, and in three months reached her ideal weight. She has stayed there for the ensuing five months. During this time she has no longer experienced the hot flashes, headaches, or sweats. As long as she continues on the medication, she should remain symptom-free.

With the data from your careful history, your thorough physical examination, your oxygen consumption tests, comprehensive laboratory tests including blood, urine, and analysis of your hair, and your electrocardiogram, I am in a position to determine exactly what's wrong with you. Why haven't you lost weight? Is there a metabolic or endocrine problem? If so, what specific treatment is necessary to correct your problem?

Then I prescribe whatever specific medication you need and construct a diet based on all my findings. From the oxygen consumption tests, I know what percent fat, carbohydrate, and protein you burn. So the diet I construct for you is specific to your needs. I then advise you on what the best exercise regimen should be—one geared for those parts of your body that need the greatest reduction, and toward the type of activities you can follow.

I know your ideal weight, I know your current weight, I know, from testing, how many calories you are burning, and I know how many calories you will be taking in on the diet I give you.

I then tell you exactly how many pounds you will lose each week until you reach your ideal weight. If you don't, the reason is that you are not following your diet. This is discussed during the follow-up visit when we talk about your nutritional diary (Chapter 6).

By following the diet, you are now on your way toward achieving your ideal weight. Once you have reached this goal, you should be reexamined to determine whether your medical problem has been corrected.

Next you want to know how to stay at your ideal weight. You gradually add back some of the foods you would like to eat. As long as you don't eat more calories than you burn, you will maintain your ideal weight.

Here's how to figure. For the first month after you have achieved your ideal weight, you should weigh yourself daily. If you gain weight on any given day, you should cut back the next day until you lose that added weight. You will then develop a balance and see how much food you can eat every day. You won't actually be counting calories, but your body will show them by the scale. You will then incorporate this into your everyday eating activities. Never allow yourself to stray more than three pounds from your ideal weight.

Q. How do you determine from your physical examination if a person has too much fat in a particular area?

A. I use a special pair of calipers to measure skin thickness. I take your skin fold and measure it with an instrument that looks like a pair of pliers with a scale on it. It is painless. This measurement will tell me if you have too much fat in different parts of your body. If you would like to approximate this test, simply pinch your skin over different parts of your body, holding it between your finger and your thumb. As a general rule for women, if you have more than a 1¼-inch skin-fold thickness, you have too much fat in that part of your body. For men, if you have a skin-fold thickness of more than 1 inch you are too fat there.

The best overall way I know to determine if you are too

fat is simply to take off all your clothes and take a good hard look at yourself in a full-length mirror. This costs nothing and will eloquently tell you the answer.

If you want to know your ideal weight and whether you need to spot reduce, Chapter 2 will give you the answers.

Q. Whom can I call to find out what doctor in my area will do the necessary tests?

A. It is always best to start with your own family doctor. If he doesn't do them he can refer you to someone who does. If he doesn't know, then you can call your local medical society and ask if there is anyone in your area who is doing work on obesity.

Q. Can fluid problems aggravate obesity?

A. Definitely. Nancy, thirty-five, a secretary for an automobile manufacturing company, was thirty-five pounds overweight. Her husband, a lawyer, says she is pleasant to live with except for the nine days before her period, when she becomes very irritable. She stays in this "miserable" state until two days after her period begins. He can time her moods by the calendar, relative to her period. Also, during this time she always regains whatever weight she had previously lost.

I thoroughly examined her and the only thing I could find was that she was too fat and had an increased amount of fluid around her ankles. She did remember always becoming excessively bloated nine days before her period. At this time her rings would get tight, her shoes would pinch, her bra would dig into her flesh, and often her face would get puffy, particularly around the eyes.

A test of her urine and blood showed she was secreting an excessive amount of a salt-retaining hormone from her adrenal gland nine days before her period. This hormone, called aldosterone, caused her to retain salt and therefore fluid. That was Nancy's problem. Previously, not realizing this, she would overeat out of disgust—because she had been gaining weight (albeit water) without overeating.

I treated Nancy with an oral medication, Aldactone, and put her on a low-salt diet. Within three months her fluid problem was completely corrected. She no longer became bloated prior to her period, nor did she any longer have the sour disposition to go along with it. Now, staying on my Easy, No-Risk Diet, she has done extremely well, losing sixteen pounds in three weeks. (It should be noted that in the medical literature there is no conclusive evidence that premenstrual fluid retention is due to an increased amount of this hormone.)

Q. It's hard to understand about the number of calories in and the number of calories out. Can you explain it simply?

A. If you eat more calories than you burn, you are going to gain weight. If you eat less calories than you burn, you will lose weight. It's that simple. You can think of it as a savings account in the bank. The number of calories you put into your mouth is analogous to the amount of money you deposit in your account. The number of calories you use (burn) each day is analogous to the amount of money you withdraw from your savings account. Your weight at any given time is analogous to the balance remaining in your account.

The ABC's of weight are simple. When calories in (A)

equal calories out (B) then your weight (C) is stable. Just as when the money you deposit (A) equals the money you withdraw (B) then your bank balance (C) does not change. On the other hand, if you eat more calories than you burn, you *must* gain weight, just as, if you deposit more money than you withdraw, your bank balance must increase. But if you eat less calories than you burn, you must lose weight. Just as, if you deposit less money than you withdraw, your bank balance must decrease.

Q. **Are there any new medical techniques that can diagnose health problems for fat people before they become crucial?**
A. Dr. Jerry Coller, an East Coast internist, believes that very thorough examining and testing can act as a prevention. For instance, using a walking electrocardiogram, he hooks his patients up to portable electrodes that are placed on their chest under their clothes. As they walk around and do their usual daily activity they are not even aware that their every heart pulse is being recorded electromagnetically. The recording continues as one sleeps, and in the morning the electrodes and tapes are taken off the chest and the records analyzed to see how the heart reacted over the previous twenty-four hours. This has the advantage over a resting electrocardiogram of showing the patient's heart reaction under all types of situations.

Most of the deaths that occur from heart disease are electrical deaths—it is not that the heart ruptures. Dr. Coller says: "Sudden death is predictable." He is the medical director for a new medispa that is being built in Florida. It will specialize in preventing people from becoming sick, with a program that will include my basic diet.

Q. Is there some general way I can determine how many calories I burn a day based on my age, weight, height and sex without going through your special test?
A. Yes. But it will be only an approximation. The following table was adapted from data by the Food and Nutrition Board, National Academy of Sciences, National Research Council. It shows you approximately the number of calories you burn up a day.

	Age	Weight– Pounds	Height– Inches	Approximate Calories Burned Per Day
Children	1	26	32	1,100
	3	35	39	1,400
	6	51	48	2,000
Boys	10	77	55	2,500
	12	95	59	2,700
	14	130	67	3,000
Girls	10	77	55	2,250
	12	97	62	2,300
	14	114	64	2,400
Men	18	147	69	2,800
	35	154	68	2,600
	55	154	67	2,400
Women	18	128	64	2,000
	35	128	63	1,850
	55	128	62	1,700

Q. I can't find myself in your table. Is there some way, having determined my ideal weight from your table in Chapter 2, that I can determine approximately the number of calories I should burn a day?
A. Yes. Take your ideal weight, and if you are a sedentary adult, multiply it by 16. That will give you the approximate

number of calories you should burn daily. If your ideal weight is 100 pounds, and you are sedentary, then multiply it by 16 and you should burn approximately 1,600 calories a day. If you are active—you do physical work or the work of a housewife—then take your ideal weight and multiply it by 20. Again, for the 100-pound person, multiplying by 20 would give you 2,000 calories to burn daily. If you are in the very active category—growing children, athletes, laborers—take your ideal weight and multiply it by 28. If your ideal weight is 100 pounds, multiplying it by 28 shows you would burn 2,800 calories a day.

Q. Do different people of the same sex, height, weight, age, and race burn approximately the same number of calories irrespective of exercise?

A. The answer is no. There is a lot of individual variation. Some people's metabolic thermostat is set high, others low. That is why the table on page 203 only gives approximations. But regardless of how many calories your body burns, you can always increase that number through exercise.

Q. Why do you think most people who lose weight but then gain it back are not successful in keeping weight off?

A. I think the majority simply revert back to their previous bad eating habits, which means that they are eating too much food. By eating more calories than they burn, they allow the pounds to creep back. The only answer is in a lifetime Figure-Keeper maintenance regimen. There are two ways you can approach this. First, if you thoroughly enjoyed my Easy, No-Risk Diet, stay on it, but add back foods you want each day. Then weigh yourself the following morning. If you gain weight, you have simply eaten too much food. Don't add as much back the next day. Keep juggling—adding and subtracting things from the basic diet until you eat just the amount of food that will keep your weight stable. If for a weekend you go away on a holiday and gain a few pounds, then as soon as you return, go back on the basic diet until you have taken off the excess weight you gained. Then add back food until you restabilize your weight.

10

UNDERSTANDING
YOUR BODY—
HOW TO STAY YOUNG
AND FIT FOR LIFE

One attitude that needs to be stamped out forever in this country is that the older you get the less valuable you are. For a society as advanced as ours, it's a pretty shortsighted point of view.

Age should be stricken from application forms, because it can be used to discriminate against you just as quickly as sex or race. All three types of discrimination are equally obnoxious. Some people are decrepit at twenty-seven. Others are not at eighty-five. The aging process begins with conception and continues throughout life.

But your individual life-style, health, diet, outlook, abilities, interests, and heredity all shape the condition you are in at any given age.

Indeed, the older person often resents the designations "golden age" or "senior citizen." If you are enjoying very good health, you may not wish to be placed in either category. Old people resent labels. Just call them by their own names.

Some of you may be middle aged, at the peak of your career and the fulfillment of your ambitions, and still have plenty of energy to burn. Others of you have retired and are enjoying a well-earned rest. And there are those who feel, as early as their sixties, that they are experiencing a decline, with increasing dependency based on their state of health, economic and social change, and loss of loved ones. It is true of all of us, however, that physical change is taking place continuously as we grow older.

Studies show that the major physiological change occurring with age is a decrease in the number of functioning cells. The cells of the liver, the stomach, and intestinal lining, skin and hair continue to divide and reproduce throughout life. Muscle and nerve cells, however, do not have this capacity, and so they gradually decrease in function. Changes occur in the connective tissue, especially collagen, which is the main supporting material in tendons, ligaments, skin, and blood vessels. As you grow older the amount of collagen changes, becoming rigid; the skin loses its flexibility, the joints creak, and the back bends. *Don't let this scare you.* While physical change does occur, it varies tremendously from person to person. You are the best judge of how fit you are. Your best protection against these changes is good nutrition and ample exercise.

I do want to run through the various processes that take place as you grow older, so that you can be aware of them and condition yourself to meet them.

Energy metabolism (the process that makes energy available to your body) also changes with age. From ages thirty to ninety your basal metabolism (minimal amount of energy used to maintain life functions) decreases by about 20 percent. There is less muscle tension and sometimes a lessening of thyroid activity. Many people find their weight increases steadily throughout their adult life, with an increasing proportion of body fat to other body tissues. This weight gain plateaus at the decade of sixty-five to seventy-four years. Thereafter a gradual decline takes place.

Undoubtedly, obesity increases susceptibility to the degenerative diseases of middle age, becomes an extra burden on weight-bearing joints, and increases the likelihood of accidents.

Because the body processes do begin to slow down, the bloodstream becomes sluggish in delivering blood, and glands produce less secretion to aid in cell function. This may account for some of the complaints of the elderly. Some may have reduced secretion of saliva and complain of dry mouth; others may experience digestive discomfort. This may be due to lowered amounts of hydrochloric acid and bile that are secreted. Problems with gas and constipation may be due to the increased activity of the stomach and decreased movement of the intestines, a common condition of older people.

Some older people gulp their food and unconsciously swallow air, which can cause great discomfort. Physical changes may also include poor teeth and gums, problems in chewing, and blunted senses of taste and smell.

The older man or woman has the same need for nutrition as the young adult—except for calories. In studies of the elderly population of the United States, it was found that many were not eating enough minerals, calcium, and iron. Also lacking in their diets were the vitamins riboflavin (B vitamins), thiamine, and ascorbic acid (vitamin C), and vitamin A.

The older person tends to follow eating patterns established in his earlier years. He has been influenced by the many factors determining food acceptance from infancy throughout life. Older people who live alone often have no incentive to cook. They may eat carbohydrate-laden foods in excess, because they are easy to chew, require little preparation, and are inexpensive. Many overlook milk because of mistaken ideas of its value for adults, its supposedly constipating or gas-producing effects, and its high cost. Fresh vegetables may be considered too difficult to chew and too expensive. Fruits are often thought to be too "acid." Many older people believe their food needs are small because they no longer have growth needs and because they are inactive.

Older people are particularly susceptible to the claims of food faddists, and spend disproportionate amounts of money on "miracle" drugs and diets. Most have limited incomes, and money should be spent wisely for nutritious food.

The individual who has had a lifetime of poor nutritional habits is not likely to be in as good health as the one who has enjoyed the benefits of a balanced diet. Good diet in later years cannot completely compensate for the years of inadequacy or correct irreversible tissue changes. It is also difficult for an older person (or anyone for that matter) to alter his whole eating pattern. Even so, the older person with unfortunate food habits who is in a poor state of nutrition can benefit greatly from following good nutritional rules applicable to all adults.

Note: This chapter does not provide information about losing weight, but gives basic nutritionally sound information for all adults.

WHAT IS GOOD NUTRITION?
FOLLOW THESE GENERAL RULES:

- *WATER* Drink 7 to 8 cups per day. This includes fluid in soup, tea, coffee, milk, juice. Many older people forget this intake. Water is necessary for good elimination, efficient kidney function, and to supply the needs of cells.
- *VITAMINS* There is much debate about the vitamin needs of the elderly. Studies show vitamin requirements do not change with age. Therefore those adequate for the young adult are the same through life. However, if the older person has a digestive problem, the need for vitamins may increase. *All the necessary vitamins are furnished by a well-balanced intake of food.* Vitamins should be taken only on the advice of the physician who will specify the amount and the kind. Much money is wasted by elderly people who feel that if a vitamin tablet is taken, all nutrient needs are satisfied! This is not true.
- *MINERALS* Here again the needs for minerals are the same as for the young adult. Since many elderly people are likely to have a deficiency of calcium and iron, a diet liberal in these minerals is suggested. Calcium is necessary for good bone mineralization throughout life. Iron is necessary to prevent anemia.
- *FIBER* Many older people select diets whose foods are smooth in character. This, together with inadequate fluid intake, can lead to persistent constipation. The fiber of tender vegetables, fruits, and whole-grain cereals will encourage normal peristalsis (intestinal movement) and bowel function. Even if they are difficult to chew or swallow, most older people can handle well-cooked vegetables and soft or stewed

210

fruits. These provide interest in the diet, are inexpensive, and are good sources of vitamins and minerals.

- *PROTEIN* This vital nutrient is found in meats, cheese, eggs, milk, beans, peas, soybeans, peanut butter, fish, and poultry. Once again, the requirement for the older person is the same as for the young adult. Because of problems of chewing and the expense of these foods, many older people skip them—a serious mistake.

  Remember this: Enough protein must be supplied each day to promote the building of cells that are destroyed each day. The meal plan (page 215) gives the amount of food necessary to supply adequate daily protein. *Also very important:* If you do not eat enough sugars and starches (carbohydrates), your body will use protein for energy needs rather than for tissue repair. How much good the protein you eat does for your body depends on the quantity and ratio of amino acids (building blocks) that the protein contains. In order to provide your body with good protein, it is estimated that one-fourth to one-half of your protein intake should come from animal sources, with the remainder derived from plant sources. If animal and plant protein foods are eaten at the same meal, you will better utilize the incomplete plant protein for tissue building. There is usually no need for supplemental amino acid preparations as some food faddists may claim. About 15 to 20 percent of the day's total calories should come from protein.

- *CARBOHYDRATES* Sugars and starches are your body's energy sources and are supplied by cereals, breads, fruits, and vegetables. Remember, carbohydrates protect the protein so that it can be used for

211

tissue repair. It is usually recommended that about 50 percent of your calories come from carbohydrate foods. Older people need to be sure their intake of carbohydrate foods is not too excessive.

- *FATS* Usually, they should contribute about 25 to 35 percent of your total calories. They provide a source of energy and supply the two essential fatty acids (ones the body needs but cannot manufacture, and therefore, that must be taken in the diet). It provides a vehicle for the fat-soluble vitamins to enter the body.

  The digestion and absorption of fats may be delayed in the older person, but there is no need to restrict fat unnecessarily. Enough fat for meal palatability aids appetite. Large portions should be avoided because of their slow absorption and increased risk of hardening of the arteries and heart problems.

- *CALORIES* Calories are obtained from fat, carbohydrate, and protein. The older person usually needs between 1,800 and 2,400 calories daily. Women over fifty require about 1,800, and men over fifty, 2,400 calories. This is because of body size and the fact that men have a difference in metabolic rate. From the eating standpoint, it's a man's world!

- *ADDITIVES* An *additive* is a substance added to food or drink in relatively small amounts to provide or improve desirable properties. Common use of additives is to make foods stay fresher longer or to suppress undesirable change such as mold or to replace vitamins and minerals lost in the processing.

  Applying the knowledge of nutrition is a complicated process. The older person can use the Basic Four Food Groups as a guide to good nutrition. Plan your menu each day to make certain you are getting adequate nutrients.

BASIC FOUR FOOD GROUPS

Dairy Foods

Milk and milk products. Milk may be dried, evaporated, fresh, or from cheeses.

One pint per day, including that used in cooking. One ounce yellow cheese may be substituted for one cup milk. Milk and milk products supply calcium.

Meat Group

Meat, fish, poultry, egg, or cheese; as alternates, dried beans, peas or nuts

Two or more servings daily (not more than four eggs per week). If you have a cholesterol or lipid problem, consult your physician for the amount of eggs you should eat.

Vegetables and Fruits

Raw, dried, cooked, frozen, or canned.

Four or more servings daily. Include a good source of ascorbic acid (vitamin C) and vitamin A.

Breads and Cereals

Natural, whole grain, or enriched

4 or more servings

Good sources of ascorbic acid (vitamin C) are oranges, grapefruits, tangerines, lemons, limes, tomatoes, and their juices; as well as strawberries, mangoes, cantaloupes, papayas, cherries, broccoli, fresh cooked turnip greens, collards, kale, cabbage family, green peppers, and potatoes with skins.

Good sources of vitamin A are leafy green vegetables, egg yolk, whole or enriched milk, butter, margarine, cream, dried fruits, apricots, canteloupe, and liver.

Additional foods are provided to satisfy appetite and energy needs.

A pattern meal plan that gives you a balanced 1,800-calorie daily intake is provided on page 215. It includes three meals and a snack. Many older people find six meals per day, using smaller quantities, more satisfactory, however. In order to ensure an adequate intake of nutrients, the amount of food in the meal plan should be eaten each day. For those older people requiring more calories, larger servings of food may be used and more desserts added, making sure the Basic Four Food Groups are included.

1,800-CALORIE MEAL PATTERN PLAN

Breakfast   1 serving fruit—remember to have a good source
of vitamin C (see Basic Four Food Groups)
1 egg any style (3 per week). Cereal may be used
instead
1 teaspoon butter or other spread
1 slice toast, 1 English muffin, biscuit, etc. (bread
shares list, page 69 through 72)
1 cup milk—skim or whole or buttermilk
Jelly or honey as desired
Coffee or tea with cream and sugar as desired

Luncheon   2 ounces meat, fish, poultry, cheese, or alternate
(see protein shares list page 64)
1 serving of vegetable
Salad if desired
2 slices of bread or substitute (see bread shares
list pages 69 through 72)
2 teaspoons of butter, spread, mayonnaise, salad
dressing
1 serving of fruit or dessert
Coffee or tea with cream and sugar as desired

Evening   3 ounces meat, fish, poultry, cheese, or alternate
Meal   (protein shares list)
2 servings of vegetables
Salad if desired
1 serving of fruit
2 slices of bread or substitute (bread shares list)
1 serving of fruit or dessert
Coffee or tea with cream and sugar as desired

Snack   1 ounce meat, fish, poultry, cheese, or alternate
1 slice of bread or substitute (bread shares list)
1 cup milk—skim, whole, or buttermilk

215

General Directions:

Meat may be broiled, roasted, stewed, braised, occasionally fried. Vegetables should be cooked in clear salted water, or simply prepared in combination with each other. Consult your favorite cookbook for interesting and new ideas. Seldom fry. One-half cup is a serving.

Fruits may be fresh, dried, frozen, or canned. Usually ½ cup is considered a serving.

Desserts may be added occasionally to the diet—not more than one a day. Servings are as follows:

> ⅛ of 9-inch pie
> ½ cup of any pudding
> 1/12 of 10-inch cake or 2-inch square
> 3 two-inch cookies

Cereal may be ¾ cup of any prepared cereal or ½ cup of cooked cereal. If unwanted weight gain occurs, cut out some desserts, use fruit without sugar, and eliminate sugar and cream from your menu plan.

The weekly menu plan found at the end of this chapter is designed for one to two persons with moderate income and limited cooking facilities. The meals are planned so that leftovers are kept to a minimum, yet variety is provided. Considerable food can be saved, if the menu is planned in advance and shopping is done accordingly. Convenience foods are kept to a minimum—only those are used that produce a saving in time and money, such as angel food cake mix. If baking facilities are not reliable, these low-calorie, delicious cakes can be purchased already baked.

Remember the Basic Four list should be used to monitor your daily food intake. Make adjustments to your own existing eating pattern if you need to. Eating is fun for you, too!

Shopping Tips

• Choose your food to meet your needs and desires.

• Foods prepared at home are usually less expensive than those partially or fully prepared. However, consider this carefully! If you must discard unused portions of food, it may be cheaper to buy partially or fully prepared foods.

• You can sometimes save money, as well as add variety to meals, if you buy small amounts of foods available in cans. Try using baby and junior foods in recipes that call for minor amounts of a vegetable or fruit. Single-serving cans, provided with snap-off lids,of beef stew, Vienna sausage, and dumplings are quick to prepare.

• Nonfat dry milk, reconstituted, is less expensive than fluid milk. It also has fewer calories than whole milk and can be made up in small amounts. You can save by mixing it half and half with fluid milk. Most people like the taste.

• Select cuts and types of meat, poultry, and fish that provide the most servings of cooked lean food for the money spent. Cuts with bone, gristle, or fat give only about half as much cooked lean meat per pound. Use leftover meat in casseroles, salads, sandwiches, soups, and as flavoring for cooked vegetables.

• Whole grain or enriched products are notably more nutritious than unenriched products, but not necessarily more expensive. Read the labels. This is particularly true of breads and cereals. Ready-to-serve cereals are usually more expensive than those you prepare yourself.

• Vegetables and fruits can be purchased fresh, frozen, canned, dried, or dehydrated. Study the cost per serving and buy in the form you can manage with your kitchen facilities.

Here are two special tips I would like to share with you:

Instant Homemade Soup

Cook vegetables in a small amount of water. Save their juice (*i.e.*, spinach, green beans, peas—you don't use it when serving vegetables). Put a bouillon cube in a cup of boiling water. Stir till dissolved. When bouillon is ready, add vegetables' juices and salt to taste. You have an instant, nutritious cup of soup. Bouillon alone is a warm and comforting drink, but is not nutritious. Or you can use this as a base for homemade vegetable soup, dicing any vegetables you like and simmering till tender. It saves the vitamins and cuts down on your grocery bill. Instead of buying cans of soup, you make soup from something you would otherwise have thrown out.

Homemade Bread

Bake your own bread—it's better and costs half as much as buying it. You'll find this recipe far less strenuous than many others. It requires *no kneading!*

Early Virginia settlers brought this from England.

> 1 package active dry yeast
> ¼ cup warm water
> 2 tablespoons vegetable shortening such as Crisco
> ½ cup sugar
> 2 eggs
> 1 teaspoon salt
> 3½ cups all-purpose flour
> 1 cup warm milk

Soften yeast in the warm water. In a mixing bowl, cream shortening and sugar. Beat in eggs and salt. Stir in 1½ cups of the flour, beat vigorously. Stir in milk and the softened yeast, mix well. Add the remaining flour, beat vigorously (use electric mixer if desired). Cover, let rise in warm place till double (about 1 hour). Stir down batter and spoon evenly into greased, 10-inch fluted tube pan or bread-loaf pan. Cover, let rise again till double (30 to 45 minutes). Bake in 325° oven for 10 minutes. Increase oven temperature to 375°, bake 20 minutes more. After cooling, remove the bread from pan. Serve warm or cool. Makes 2 loaves. Delicious with cinnamon and sugar. Slice. Toast one side; butter the other. Sprinkle already mixed cinnamon and sugar on buttered side. Place buttered side up in broiler.

Living Alone

Q. You no longer cook for a family, and it doesn't seem worthwhile to prepare a big dinner for one person. What do you do?

A. Go right ahead and cook as if for one big family. Eat your single portion of everything. Then, put the remainder in TV dinner aluminum trays—each in its own space—and store three, four, five dinners in the freezer. You don't have to cook every day. Just take out your homemade TV dinners and pop in the oven.

If you would like to stay young and fit as you grow older, then *good nutrition is a must.* I have prepared the following week's menu plan for you. It is just an example. You can design your own plan to fit your particular needs.

Suggested Week of Balanced, Nutritious Menus

Monday

Breakfast ½ cup orange juice
1 egg poached on toast with 1 teaspoon butter
½ cup milk
Coffee or tea as desired, with sugar and cream

Lunch Grilled cheese sandwich
Tomato wedges on lettuce with salad dressing
Canned peaches
1 cup milk
Coffee or tea if you wish

Dinner 3 ounces meatloaf
½ cup mashed potato
½ cup green peas
Tossed green salad with favorite dressing
½ cup chocolate pudding
Coffee or tea if you wish

Snack 1 cup milk
1 slice cheese
5 saltine crackers

Tuesday

Breakfast   ½ grapefruit
¾ cup cornflakes
1 cup milk
1 slice toast with 1 teaspoon butter or other
spread
Jelly if desired
Coffee or tea as you like it

Lunch   1 hard-cooked egg sliced on 1 tablespoon of tuna,
chopped green pepper on ½ English muffin with
⅓ cup hot cheese soup over the tuna
Celery sticks
1 cup milk
1 fresh or baked apple
Coffee or tea as you wish

Dinner   1 broiled chicken breast
½ cup scalloped potatoes
Broccoli spears
Peaches in jello
Dinner roll with butter or spread
Coffee or tea as you wish

Snack   1 cup milk
1 tablespoon peanut butter
1 slice bread

221

Wednesday

Breakfast ½ cup orange juice
½ cup cream of wheat with sugar
1 English muffin with butter or spread
½ cup milk
Jelly if desired
Coffee or tea as you like it

Lunch Meatloaf sandwich
Lettuce wedge with salad dressing
1 cup milk
1 banana
Coffee or tea as you wish

Dinner Tuna noodle casserole or tuna patty
½ cup green beans
Coleslaw
Dinner roll or bread with butter or spread
Angel food cake
Coffee or tea as you wish

Snack ¾ cup prepared cereal
1 cup milk
Sugar as desired

Thursday

Breakfast   ½ grapefruit
½ cup oatmeal
1 cup milk
1 slice toast or 1 English muffin
1 teaspoon butter or spread
Jelly as desired
Coffee or tea

Lunch   French toast with powdered sugar
Cottage cheese on lettuce
Pineapple slices
½ cup milk
Coffee or tea

Dinner   Baked pork chop
½ cup mashed potato
Broccoli spears
Spicy applesauce
1 slice bread and 1 teaspoon butter
½ cup chocolate pudding
Coffee or tea

Snack   1 cup milk
1 tablespoon peanut butter
or 1 slice Angel Food Cake
2 graham crackers or 5 saltines

223

Friday

Breakfast   ½ cup orange juice
1 egg, scrambled
1 slice toast
1 teaspoon butter or spread
½ cup milk
Jelly if desired
Coffee or tea

Lunch   Creamed chipped beef on toast
Green beans
Apple salad
Ice cream
Coffee or tea

Dinner   Hamburger patty on bun
Coleslaw, or lettuce wedge, if you prefer
1 cup milk
1 slice angel food cake
Coffee or tea

Snack   1 cup milk
¾ cup prepared cereal
Sugar if desired

Saturday

Breakfast   ½ grapefruit
½ cup oatmeal
1 cup milk
1 slice toast or 1 English muffin
1 teaspoon butter or spread
Coffee or tea

Lunch   Cheese soup
Peanut butter and bacon sandwich
Cucumber and tomato slices salad with dressing
1 cup milk
2 pineapple slices
Coffee or tea

Dinner   Broiled flounder filet with lemon butter
½ cup creamed potato
½ cup green peas
Lettuce heart with salad dressing
Dinner roll or 1 slice bread with butter or spread
Baked apple

Snack   1 cup milk
1 slice cheese
1 slice bread   } can run under broiler

Sunday

Breakfast   1 orange, sliced
1 egg, fried
2 slices bacon if desired
1 slice toast
1 teaspoon butter or spread
½ cup milk
Coffee or tea

Lunch   Cottage cheese on lettuce with fruit
Toasted English muffin or bread
1 cup milk
Angle food cake
Coffee or tea as desired

Dinner   1 slice broiled ham
½ cup creamed potato
Green beans
Broiled peach half
Dinner roll or 1 slice bread
1 teaspoon butter or spread
Ice cream
Coffee or tea as desired

Snack   1 cup milk
2 graham crackers

11

THE BYPASS—

THE OPERATION THAT

GUARANTEES QUICK

WEIGHT LOSS

You're not just fat. You're obese. *Morbidly obese.* You have trouble walking, working, buying clothes, even doing such everyday things as going to the toilet and taking a bath. You have tried dieting and failed. You may have lost more than 100 pounds, but gained it back. You're in a real state of emergency. What can you do?

Q. What is "morbid obesity"?
A. Physicians apply this term to massively obese people whose health and life are actually threatened by their overweight state. These are people who weigh two to three times their ideal weight.

Q. What is the intestinal bypass operation?
A. For the last twenty years, surgeons have been performing and perfecting the intestinal bypass operation. The

patient's intestinal tract—normally twenty-one feet long—is shortened to eighteen to twenty-four inches. As a result of the shortened gastrointestinal (GI) tract, much less food is absorbed into the body; therefore, although the patient continues to eat a lot, and does not diet, he loses weight rapidly. The part of the intestine not being used is reconnected and drained into the small intestine for safe-keeping in case the patient needs to be reconnected at a later time. In short, the operation allows him to eat as much as he desires and lose weight at the same time. Patients usually lose 100 to 150 pounds in the first twelve to eighteen months, depending on how fat they are to begin with, and then level off at a plateau that is still above their ideal weight.

Dr. H. William Scott, Jr., Professor and Chairman, Department of Surgery, Vanderbilt University Medical Center, Nashville, reported the case of a twenty-seven-year-old farmer who weighed 350 pounds and had been overweight all his life. He had tried many different forms of dieting—all unsatisfactorily. His mother was very heavy but his father was not. His obesity problem was complicated by a high proportion of lipids (fatty substances) in his blood which increased his risk of heart disease.

"When, moreover, the patient is psychologically incapable of following dietary and exercise advice, the physician has only two realistic choices," Dr. Scott observed. "He can abandon hope or he can contemplate a surgical approach to the problem."

The farmer underwent the bypass operation, was discharged from the hospital ten days later, and within a month had lost forty-eight pounds. His weight was expected to stabilize twelve to eighteen months later.

Dr. Scott also reported in the medical literature that twelve patients who underwent his modified form of the Payne-

DeWind bypass operation averaged losing 31 percent of their body weight within twenty months after their operations.

Q. Can anyone who is fat and tired of dieting have the operation?
A. No. There are some risks involved, and leading medical centers as well as trustworthy private surgeons have adopted certain criteria for candidates for the operation. Dr. J. Howard Payne and Dr. Loren T. DeWind of the University of Southern California School of Medicine in Los Angeles, pioneers in the intestinal bypass, adopted these requirements:
—The candidate must be at least 125 pounds overweight
—all other nonsurgical reducing methods have failed
—life is endangered by a disease such as the Pickwickian Syndrome (excessively fat people who because of their fatness don't breathe properly and readily fall asleep while talking to you), diabetes (increased sugar in your blood), or hypertension (high blood pressure).

At Johns Hopkins Hospital, in Baltimore, the operation is reserved for patients who are:
—age 15–45 years
—100–125 percent overweight
—proven diet failures
—seemingly good candidates psychologically as determined by a psychiatric evaluation

The first patient to receive the bypass at Johns Hopkins was a 6 foot 4 inch seventeen-year-old boy who weighed 528 pounds. He had quit high school at the end of his sophomore year when he was fifteen. "We had to see him in the parking lot because he was ashamed to walk through the hospital," recalled Dr. Dean Lockwood, an endocrinologist who oversees the bypass program at Johns Hopkins.

Now twenty-one, the patient weights about 235 pounds— less than half his former weight.

Johns Hopkins has performed seventy bypass operations in the last three years. Two of the patients died. One died from halothane hepatitis—allergic reactions to anesthesia—within five weeks of the surgery. The other died from liver disease.

Q. How great are the risks in the bypass and just what are they?

A. The biggest risk is liver failure. However, under the type of close medical follow-up care that now exists at Johns Hopkins, Vanderbilt, Southern California, University of Maryland, and other hospitals where physicians have a planned bypass program, this does not have to be a reason not to have the operation. With regular liver biopsies (examining liver tissue), adequate supplemental vitamins and careful, tender loving care long after the operation, liver failure can be avoided. If it develops, it can be detected early enough to treat.

At worst, if you *do* show symptoms of a failing liver and do not respond to medical treatment, the surgeon can hook you back up. No portion of your intestine was cut off and thrown away in the bypass operation. Therefore, if the need arises, your intestinal tract can be rejoined to its full length.

Q. Why might liver failure occur?

A. For two reasons. First, an inexperienced surgeon could cut too short a segment, resulting in inadequate nutrition. The intestine is like an accordion, and is difficult to measure exactly. Yet precise measurement is crucial to this operation. Second, if you receive poor follow-up care, or none at all—your warning signs of liver disorder could go unnoticed until too late. Signals could be excessive tiredness, swelling, leg cramps, unaccounted for black and blue marks, nausea and vomiting. Those yards of intestine protect the liver, and after the digestive process no longer includes this long route, the liver could get a lot of abuse from very poisonous substances.

If you don't eat enough protein, your liver can become chock full of fats and you can subsequently develop fibrosis which is replacement of your functioning liver tissue with non-functioning scar tissue. A fatty liver frequently corrects itself when your weight stabilizes and is usually prevented by eating a well-balanced, nutritionally sound diet. You particularly need to eat adequate amounts of protein.

The fibrosis can also be stopped by reconnecting the intestine and eating a nutritionally sound diet.

Q. Are there any other problems associated with the operation?
A. Yes. High on the list is diarrhea, which is usually severe for the first one to three months. You may have six to ten semisolid stools a day, or even more. When the condition levels off, you have a minimum of two to five movements a day. They may be very smelly because food taken in has been malabsorbed (not adequately digested and absorbed into the body). Diarrhea can be controlled somewhat with medicines.

Close on the heels of diarrhea can come proctitis (inflammation of the rectum) and hemorrhoids. Chemicals (bile acids) in the diarrhea which normally are absorbed in the ileum no longer are, and therefore cause a continuing irritation. You know this because your rectum feels sore.

Your doctor can give you medicine to alleviate some or all of the soreness. You may occasionally lose a few days work because of these highly annoying problems.

A third unfortunate side effect of the bypass is a tendency toward vitamin and mineral deficiencies. This, too, can be remedied.

A small percentage of patients get gallstones (6 percent) or kidney stones (8 percent), according to Dr. Lockwood. Some patients experience increased uric acid which can lead to gout.

Q. After the operation can you continue to eat and drink anything you want?

A. "In view of the danger of liver failure, alcohol in the first year is an absolute no," advises Dr. T. Brannon Hubbard, Jr., professor of surgery at University Hospital in Maryland, who is experienced in the bypass. Fatty and greasy foods will cause more diarrhea, he says.

Q. What are the positive effects of the bypass?

A. Most important to the patient who submitted to the operation is the rapid weight loss that results automatically. Patients tend to lose about one-third of their total weight.

Most patients lose to this far safer weight level, then stabilize their weight and do not have to have their intestinal tracts hooked back together. Although they don't have to worry about counting calories, many patients find their appetites change and old cravings diminish or vanish.

In addition to feeling better physically, patients who have lost weight after the bypass talk about how much better they feel psychologically. A handicap like morbid obesity can affect you "across the board" in your social activities, sex life, work, dress, and on and on.

One forty-one-year-old woman who had the bypass after she tipped the scales at 350 pounds, in July, 1972, said seventeen months later, "It's a miracle. I ate myself into being a diabetic," Ellen reminisced over a cup of tea in her kitchen. She had remarried in 1970. "I had trouble with my periods. I had trouble with my sex life." She was employed either as a saleslady or in a clothing factory, and had trouble working, walking, or standing.

All her five aunts weighed over 300 pounds, but she said her mother had never had a weight problem. Ellen was a chubby child, and for the last twenty years had been what she termed "heavy." "I think I ate for comfort because I was an insecure child," she said. "My father died at an early age, and I loved him dearly."

Over the years, she tried diet after diet, but never managed to stay on one. Finally, extremely depressed, she went to a ten-week psychosomatic clinic at Johns Hopkins to try to find out why she could not follow a diet. While there she learned of the bypass operation. She read all the literature she could find about it. Six months later she made her decision.

"God, what have I done to myself?" she thought when she woke up from the operation.

But a year and a half later, despite bouts of diarrhea as often as fifteen to twenty times a day during the first seven weeks, and then tapering off to three to five times daily, painful hemorrhoids, and "some bad vitamin deficiencies," Ellen is very glad she had the bypass. She continues under regular medical supervision and says she feels better now than before the operation.

"If you can go out on the street and get whistled at by a

man when you haven't been whistled at in twenty years—it's quite a feeling.''

Another beneficial side effect is that all intestinal bypass patients sustain low cholesterol in their blood—which helps the heart and arteries do their job well.

My own recommendation: This operation should only be resorted to as the final step in your fight to control your weight and live a fuller, longer life. Be very careful that the surgeon you pick is experienced and qualified to perform this particular operation. Equally important is to know in advance that a medical doctor will follow your progress for months and even years after the operation, giving such supportive aid as is necessary.

A national intestinal bypass club has been formed by David Smoeller from Pikesville, Maryland, who successfully underwent the operation in July, 1972, when he was twenty-six. His weight subsequently dropped from 375 pounds to 225 pounds in December, 1973.

David, who owns two orthopedic shops, went back to work one week after leaving the hospital. He started the National Bypass Organization, Inc.,* in order "to promote a better understanding of the operation and make the recipients more aware of what will happen pre- and post- op (before and after the operation).'' For David, the bypass worked well. "It's changed my life considerably,'' he says. "I went from a twenty-two-inch (neck) to a sixteen-and-one-half shirt, and fifty-six-inch waist pants to thirty-eight. I'm living a normal life today—completely normal in every

*National Small Bowel Bypass Organization, Inc.
1707 Covington St.
Baltimore, Maryland 21230
Phone 301-837-1327

way." He summed up his feelings and probably those of many others who have new bodies because of the bypass:

"I'm under a great deal less pressure. I don't have to go to bed at night and be afraid I'm going to die. I don't have to worry that a friend of mine is picking me up in a sports car. I don't have to worry that when I walk down the street little kids are going to laugh at me."

12

INSTANT

SPOT REDUCTION

THROUGH COSMETIC SURGERY—

THE PROS AND

CONS

Instant spot reducing is also possible through surgery. But it too should be reserved for patients who are grossly obese and carrying their excess fat in particular places. For instance, an apron of fat hanging down over your genitals can be uncomfortable, make it difficult for you to clean yourself, and awkward to have sexual intercourse. If repeated diets and exercise geared to spot reduction have failed, then you may be a candidate for the plastic surgeon.

Plastic surgery can also tighten up hanging skin and wrinkling caused by rapid weight loss. Exercise can only correct a small amount of the wrinkling.

These operations can literally and figuratively change your life.

These are the fat operations most commonly done:

Eyelids. Rarely done for obesity because they don't tend to get fat. Usually eyelid surgery is a tightening technique done as an adjunct to the face-lift, especially for the patient who has lost a lot of weight. It may make you look five years younger or just more rested and refreshed. You can have it done as an outpatient, or some surgeons prefer to keep you hospitalized for two days. Swelling around the eyes usually persists for forty-eight hours—itching for up to four days. When you go outside during the first two weeks after the operation, you should wear dark glasses. The eyelid operation costs between $500 and $1,000.

Face-lift. Directed at cheeks and neck, it can include correction of an unattractive, wattled, turkey-gobbler neck. The incision is generally in the temple hair, in front of the hair and across the mastoid (behind the ear). Excess skin is then cut away from the underlying area and the remainder is pulled back.

This operation is not too effective in people who do not have a crease in their neck unless the surgeon first removes some fat from underneath the chin and accentuates the neck crease. The positive effects of the operation usually last for three to seven years. Then you can repeat it. Most people who have the face-lift operation lose weight during the first week after the operation because they are not eating well—usually beginning on a liquid diet, progressing to pureed foods and then to a soft diet. Arrange to have your face-lift at a time when you don't have too many important things to talk about, because you should refrain from abundant talking during the week following the operation.

Hospitalization: three to five days for face-lift and adjunct neck surgery.

Recovery period: two to three weeks. Bruising is the main problem, but there is little discomfort except for pain around your ears which lasts for about seventy-two hours.

Fee: About $2,500

At a later date, when the bruising has disappeared, the surgeon can do an adjunct to the face-lift called a face peel, to get rid of fine wrinkles. The face is painted with a chemical that produces a controlled second-degree burn and swelling. You will experience a sharp, stinging pain which lasts for about fifteen minutes. You will then have a feeling of facial discomfort that lasts for about five days. Again you will be on a liquid and soft diet, and will need to restrict talking for about one week. You will probably have an uncomfortable scab for about a week. *It is important to stay out of the sun for six months after the face peel.* If you don't, the ultraviolet from the sun can cause you to become unevenly hyperpigmented (increased coloration of the skin).

The peel is usually done on an outpatient basis, although some doctors prefer to keep you hospitalized for seventy-two hours. The cost is between $250 to $1,000.

Arms. When your skin hangs like a cape, it can be cut away. Here the scar that is necessary will run from the elbow to the armpit and is probably worth the improvement. It's a visible scar, running up the back of the arm, but it's somewhat less unattractive to many women than the wing of fat appearance. Although a scar can be diminished, it cannot be removed by plastic surgery. Anything that goes through the dermis (deep layer of the skin) results in a permanent scar. Lower animals will regenerate new skin, erasing a scar, but humans have lost that ability. A scar can however be modified. Fat and extra skin are simply cut away, and the opening closed. If, as you hold your arms straight out, large wings of skin flap between your elbow and your shoulder, then you are a candidate for the operation. Fee: About $1,000 for both arms. Hospitalization: three days.

Breasts. This operation is called reduction mammoplasty. It is to reduce the size of too-large breasts. The surgeon is a sculptor, and it is a major operation. The patient loses a fair amount of blood and may need a blood transfusion on the table. Usually the patient comes in a week ahead of time and gives blood, so that her own blood will be available. For any elective operation, many people are becoming their own donors. It is the safest—no fear of hepatitis (liver disease). The operation lasts from two to four hours. The surgeon might remove as much as twelve pounds in an operation like this. There are two methods: On older patients, the surgeon is more apt to do a nipple grafting procedure. If the nipple has to be raised more than five inches, most surgeons will do it as a graft. If under five inches, as a direct transplant. The main difference in the two types of operations is whether the nipple is left attached to the ducts and brought up, or whether the nipple is severed and reattached after the breast has been cut down and molded to proper proportion. Patients before the operation have complained of big red raw areas under their breasts, areas that are hard to keep clean, and pain in their back and neck. X-ray has shown a bra strap actually had left grooves in their bones.

For the first forty-eight hours after the reduction mammoplasty operation you are likely to have significant pain and discomfort. This gradually disappears by the end of the first week. You have to remember to restrict arm movement from going above your head and lifting anything heavier than a purse for about three weeks. You will probably also be wearing a special bra for almost a month. During this time your mate should not fondle your newly formed breasts. Hospitalization: Five to seven days. Cost: $1,000 to $2,000.

Abdomen. Varies from person with a small pouch to one with a big apron. The apron hanging down over the genitals can be uncomfortable and make it hard to keep yourself clean. The major belly lift is the most formidable of obese operations. It may involve pulleys on the ceiling with wires lifting up the apron during surgery. The apron might weigh from thirty to forty pounds. The patient may lose a tremendous amount of blood and may require hypotensive anesthesia. One Mexican surgeon has developed a spit he turns patients on, cutting and sewing as the patient rotates. A big apron operation lasts from two to six hours. You will be out of commission for about four weeks. For the first ten days after surgery, you will experience pain on movement and bending. By the end of the first month, though, the pain generally subsides.

The benefits range from cosmetic—looking good in a bathing suit—to doing away with a moist, smelly, discolored area under your abdominal crease. It also corrects excessive wrinkling of the belly. Hospitalization: One to two weeks. Cost: $1,000 to $2,500.

Thighs. Before surgery the fatty thigh folds often result in persistent irritation, often causing a red, hot, moist, odorous crease. The skin in this area can break down and cause ulceration. The surgeon removes a band of tissue around the upper thigh in the crease of the buttocks and up through the groin and buttocks. This operation has great cosmetic benefits. You no longer need be embarrassed by those huge, bulging thighs. After the operation you can expect to be chaste for about three to six weeks. Hospitalization: One week. Cost: $1,500 to $2,500.

Buttocks. This operation can be done in concert with the thigh operation or separately. The surgeon simply takes out excess fat overhanging your buttocks. The benefits range from purely cosmetic—looking better in a bathing suit—to improving your body hygiene by permitting you to cleanse yourself adequately.

You will be in the hospital for about one week, but it will take you about three weeks until you will be able to move your body freely during exercise. Cost: $1,000 to $2,000.

Elephantiasis. An operation for people who have massive-ly swollen legs due to blockage of the lymphatics (vessels that drain lymph fluid). Often the skin will become taut, discolored, and break down with a skin ulcer. The surgeon cuts out the excess fat and blocked lymphatic vessels. He then skin grafts down to the leg muscle. The operation will provide relief from the ulceration and will allow the deep lymphatics of the leg to drain away the lymph fluid. The leg will still remain big but not as grotesquely large as it was previously.

Expect to be in the hospital from one to three weeks. The cost of the operation is from $1,500 to $3,000.

Q. What are the possible complications of operations for obesity?

A. The same as in any surgery—infection, blood clots collecting in the wound, sluffing of tissue, loss of blood supply. Also, the problem with obese patients is that they do not have a good blood supply in their skin. This makes them very susceptible to infection and a condition called fat neutrosis in which fat undergoes spontaneous dissolution and forms an abscess in the wound.

Also, when a nerve is cut off, a small, painful tumor can develop, though it is very unusual. Severing of certain nerves can cause loss of movement. But this is also very rare. The surgeon has to be careful in a face-lift not to sever a nerve that will cause paralysis of the lower lip. But in general, the vast majority of patients I interviewed believed that the cosmetic benefit, coupled with their positive psychological lift, outweighed the side effects of plastic surgery. Most patients were happy after the operation because they knew they were doing something for themselves—improving themselves—and that was a positive feeling.

Q. How do you choose a plastic surgeon?
A. Ask your family doctor or call the local Medical Society and request the names of the board-certified surgeons. Or ask a friend who is happy with his or her surgical result. There are specialists in certain areas of the body, but they are few and far between, and not always the best.

"A specialist is a man who only does one thing and an expert is one who does something well, but may do many things," one plastic surgeon advised.

Q. Can a patient order his own operation?
A. "There are plastic surgeons who will work as technicians, and you can come and order what you want and they'll do it, and there are plastic surgeons who are physicians and you can come and they will accept you as a patient and look at you in totality and advise you of what you could have done and tell you what the possible drawbacks are and help you make up your mind whether or not you want it. And then farther over there's the physician who's God, and he will say: 'Thou shalt have or thou shalt not' and there will be no discussion and he will only take good candidates and he rejects many people," the same surgeon, who requested anonymity, replied.

"I've seen many people who have gone to see very well known surgeons and have been thrown out of their offices because they weren't very good candidates for surgery," he added. "But they were left completely mystified as to why they were or weren't operated on. Medicine's a heavy ego food and the doctor has his problems just like the patient."

The material for this chapter was drawn from interviews with various renowned plastic surgeons across the country.

13

ARE YOU

TOO THIN? WOULD

YOU LIKE A DIET

TO GAIN

WEIGHT?

"Hey, skinny—a good wind would blow you over!" These insensitive words were what brought Pete, a seventeen-year-old high school senior from Akron, to see if we could find out why he was so thin and could not gain weight.

After taking a careful history, a thorough physical examination, and the appropriate diagnostic laboratory tests, I determined that Pete was one of the few people who did have a bona fide medical reason for being thin. His thyroid gland was overactive, causing him to burn over 6,500 calories a day. Since it was highly unlikely that he would ever eat 6,500 calories a day, it is no wonder he had trouble maintaining his weight, let alone gaining weight. He was treated with proper medication to bring his thyroid to normal and put on a gaining diet. In six months he put on the thirty-two pounds he was underweight, and he has held onto it for three years.

The only way you can gain weight is to eat more calories than you burn.

Carol was a twelve-year-old girl from Los Angeles who was sixteen pounds underweight. Thorough examination showed she had no metabolic problem that caused her to burn an abnormally high number of calories. All she needed to do was to eat more. We gave her a diet loaded with food, but particularly the foods she enjoyed eating and it took her two months to pick up the sixteen pounds. She has now been at her ideal weight, eating normally for the last two years.

With 20 percent of the population in the United States frankly obese, the person who has the opposite problem is seldom considered. The thin man or woman in the minority finds a dearth of advice on how to round out the angles. Some body fat is needed to support the organs, circulatory system, and nervous system. There are some people who for health reasons *need* to gain weight.

If you are too thin, you should consult your physician to determine the amount of weight you should gain for your particular body type. Your doctor will also ferret out any *physical* reason for thinness.

If you don't have a causative medical problem, then gaining pounds is a much slower process than shrinking them off. You will want to set attainable goals of one-half to one pound per week. A slow, steady weight gain provides you with an easier adjustment of body size. Be prepared to alter clothing to avoid a pinched, stuffed feeling. Be prepared for a new wardrobe eventually, depending on the amount of weight to be gained. Your body needs to adjust to the increased food intake. Body weight may fluctuate daily due to water balance. True weight gain is evident when you weigh once weekly at the same time before dressing in the morning.

This diet allows you to gear eating to your own schedule. But, remember—skipping meals and irregular meal hours do not contribute to weight gain.

The National Institute of Health recommends that individuals prone to heart disease (your physician can advise you—yes, some thin people have elevated fats in their blood such as cholesterol and triglycerides) change the type and amount of fat used. Of particular concern are saturated fats and cholesterol. Although your diet is moderate in fat, you may wish to change the type of fat used. If your physician feels you need to modify the fat in your intake, use vegetable oils and soft margarines rich in polyunsaturated fats in place of butter and other cooking fats that are solid or hydrogenated. Read the labels. Further instructions appear on pages 89 through 90).

GENERAL INSTRUCTIONS FOR
SIMPLE WEIGHT GAIN DIET

Use the amounts of food listed. You may eat more if you wish. However, you may initially need to force yourself to include the amount specified.

Meats may be baked, broiled, or roasted. Any seasoning, gravy, or cream sauce, to make the meat more appetizing, may be used.

Vegetables may be cooked in any way you desire. Invest a little in cookbooks for exciting ways to enhance these interesting foods. Have a serving of green or yellow vegetables to insure adequate intake of vitamin A.

Have a serving of oranges, tomotoes, grapefruits, cantaloupe, or strawberries each day to provide adequate ascorbic acid (vitamin C). Raw broccoli, raw cabbage, collards, kale, and freshly cooked turnip greens are also good sources.

Desserts are an excellent way of assimilating hidden calories in concentrated form. The fruits, vegetables, meats, and dairy and cereal products will provide adequate minerals and vitamins, proteins and fats, and carbohydrates. Be sure to eat at least as many desserts as are specified in the diet.

Plan your meals ahead so that you can be sure the amount of food required by the diet is on hand.

Always eat sitting at a table. Eat slowly and chew your food well. If you are inclinced to eat fast, slow down. Be sure your fluid intake is equal to six to eight glasses of water daily.

It is important to eat at least three meals daily, spaced about four or five hours apart. *Breakfast is a must.* Some people find it easier to increase their calorie intake by having six small meals. Others find three meals with a snack results in better weight gain. Experiment and find which method suits you best. *But always eat the amount of food specified in the meal plan.* If you don't gain weight on this plan, eat even more.

Don't forget exercise. If you are inclined to skip meals when tension builds, try some form of exercise to work off stress.

If you smoke, stop. Not only will this improve your health, but you will also gain weight. Substitute food for cigarettes. A dried prune instead of a cigarette is highly recommended.

EASY, WEIGHT-GAIN DIET
(2,400–3,000 calories)

SEVEN OR MORE PROTEIN SERVINGS

THREE SERVINGS OF FRUIT

FOUR OR MORE BREAD SERVINGS

TWO OR MORE VEGETABLE SERVINGS

TWO OR MORE SERVINGS OF CEREAL AND VEGETABLE
STARCHES

ONE PINT OF MILK

ONE TEASPOON JAM, JELLY, PRESERVES, HONEY,
MOLASSES, SYRUP

ONE OR MORE SERVINGS OF DESSERT

ONE OR MORE WEIGHT-GAINING SNACK

Follow the pattern meal plan for seven days, and then add a snack from the Easy, Weight-Gaining Snack List. This may be taken in midafternoon or evening, but it must be consumed each day. A thick milk shake made with plenty of ice cream is a great snack. If weight gain does not occur, increase food intake. The food lists tell you the *minimum* size of serving to be eaten.

The snack should be eaten at the time of day that does not interfere with the amount of food scheduled to be eaten at mealtime. Determine your appetite pattern by using a daily diary (see Chapter 6).

EASY, WEIGHT-GAIN PATTERN MEAL PLAN
BREAKFAST
1 serving of fruit (see weight-gaining lists, pages 252 through 259)
1 serving cereal—any hot or dry cereal (see list)
1 to 2 eggs prepared any style
1 to 2 bread shares
1 teaspoon jelly, jam, preserves, honey, molasses
1 cup milk
Coffee or tea as desired
NOON
3–4 ounces of meat or 3–4 protein shares (see list)
2 bread shares
2 or more fat shares (see list)
Vegetable or salad
Dessert or fruit (see list)
1 cup milk
Coffee or tea as desired, cream and sugar as desired
MIDAFTERNOON
Weight-gaining snack—if this is best for you
P.M.
3–4 ounces of meat or 3–4 protein shares
1 or more serving potatoes, noodles, rice (see list of vegetable starches)
1 serving vegetable or salad
1 bread share
2 fat shares
Dessert (see list)
Coffee or tea with cream and sugar as desired
EVENING
Weight-gaining snack—if this is best for you

If you are eating more than the pattern meal plan, do not decrease your intake of food. Change it to match the pattern meal plan, so that you are eating three to six meals each day, and add more weight-gaining snacks.

WEIGHT-GAINING MILK SHARES

	Measure
Milk, evaporated	½ cup
Milk, powdered, reconstituted	1 cup
Buttermilk	1 cup
Milk	1 cup
Yogurt made with whole milk	1 cup

WEIGHT-GAINING PROTEIN SHARES

Each one contains 7 grams of protein, 5 grams of fat (75 calories)

	Measure
Meat and poultry (moderate fat) (beef, lamb, pork, liver, etc.)	1 ounce
Cold cuts (4½ inches square, ⅛ inch thick)	1 slice
Frankfurters (8–9 pounds)	1
Fish	1 ounce
Salmon, tuna, crab, lobster	¼ cup
Oysters, shrimp, clams	5
Sardines (well drained)	3
Cheese, Cheddar and American	1 ounce
Cottage cheese	¼ cup
Egg	1
Peanut butter	2 tablespoons

WEIGHT-GAINING FRUIT SHARES

Fresh, frozen, dried, canned

	Measure
Apple	1
Apple juice	⅔ cup
Applesauce	¾ cup
Apricots (dried) or candied, canned	6/2
Apricots (fresh)	2 medium
Banana	1

*Berries (black, raspberries, and strawberries)	1 cup
Blueberries (fresh or water-packed)	⅔ cup
*Cantaloupe	½ (6-inch diam.)
Cherries (Bing)	15 large
Cherries (Royal Anne)	15
Dates	6
Figs	3 large
Figs (dried)	1 small
Fruit cocktail	¾ cup
*Grapefruit	½
*Grapefruit juice	¾ cup
*Grapefruit sections	⅔ cup
Grapes	24 large, at least
Grapes (seedless)	36 small
Grape juice	1 cup
Guava	1
*Honeydew melon	⅓ (7-inch diam.)
*Mango	1 medium
Nectarine	2 medium
*Orange	1 medium
*Orange juice	¾ cup
*Orange (mandarin)	1½ cups
*Papaya	½ medium
Peach	1 large or 2 halves, canned
Pear	1 large or 2 halves, canned
Pineapple (fresh or water-packed)	¾ cup
Pineapple	2 slices
Pineapple juice	⅔ cup
Plantain	1½ inch long slice
Plums	2 large
Prune juice	½ cup
Prunes (dried)	4 medium
Raisins	4 tablespoons
*Tangerine	1 large
*Tomato juice	1 cup
Watermelon (without rind)	1½ cups
Watermelon (with rind)	1 round, 1 inch thick

*Good source of vitamin C, have a serving each day

WEIGHT-GAINING VEGETABLE SHARES

Fresh or frozen, cooked in salted water, canned. Prepared any style, creamed, scalloped, fried. Have at least ½ cup to ¾ cup as a serving.

Vegetables contain little carbohydrate, protein, or calories, and are rich in vitamins and minerals. Have a serving of a green or yellow vegetable each day for vitamin A.

Asparagus	Lettuce
Beet greens	Mushrooms
Beets	*Mustard greens
*Broccoli	Okra
*Brussels sprouts	Onion
*Cabbage (all kinds)	Oyster plant
Carrots	Parsnips
Cauliflower	Peas (green)
Celery	Poke
Chard	Pumpkin
Chicory	Radishes
*Collards	Rutabagas
Corn	Sauerkraut
Cucumber	Spinach
Dandelion greens	Summer squash
Eggplant	Tomatoes
Endive	Turnip greens
Escarole	Turnips
Green beans	Watercress
Kale	Wax beans
Kohlrabi	Winter squash
Leeks	

*Good sources of vitamin C

Each item contains 5 grams of fat (45 calories). Use as much as you like, but plan at least the amount listed.

Avocado (4-inch diameter)	⅛
Bacon (crisp)	1 slice
Butter or margarine	1 teaspoon
Cream cheese	1 tablespoon
Cream, heavy (32 percent butterfat)	1 tablespoon
Cream, light (18 percent butterfat)	2 tablespoons
French dressing	1 tablespoon
Mayonnaise	1 teaspoon
Nuts	6 small
Oil or cooking fat	1 teaspoon
Olives (ripe)	5 small
Olives (green)	10 medium
Cream, sour	2 tablespoons

Fat has great satiety value and can act as an appetite depressant. If your appetite is fleeting, use only the amount listed in the pattern meal plan.

WEIGHT-GAINING BREAD AND BREAD SHARES

Bagel	1
Biscuit (2-inch diam.)	2
Bread, enriched, whole grain, raisin	1
Cornbread (2 inches sq., 1 inch thick)	1
Muffin (small)	2
Muffin, english	1
Pancake (4-inch diam.)	2
Roll, dinner small	2
hamburger or hard	1
hot dog	1
Tortilla (6-inch diam.)	2
Waffle (5-inch diam.)	1

CAKES AND COOKIES
UNICED

Angel food (12 slices per cake)	1 piece
Plain, (mix 12 pieces per cake)	1 piece
Pound (1-inch slice)	1
Doughnuts, (plain, raised or cake type)	1–2
Chocolate chip	2–4
Fruitana raisin	1–4
Ginger or lemon snaps	5–10
Oatmeal	1–3
Pop-ups	1–2
Sugar	1–2
Vanilla Wafers	6–8

CEREALS AND VEGETABLE STARCHES

Cereal (cooked)	¾ cup
Cereal (dry: flake or puffed)	¾ cup
Corn (large ear)	½ cup
Dried beans and peas (cooked)	1 cup
Grits, rice, noodles, spaghetti	¾ cup
Potatoes:	Baked white (2-inch diam.) 1 med. to large
French fries, frozen	2 ounces
Mashed, boiled	¾ cup
Puffs (frozen—small pkg.)	½
Sweet or yam	¾ cup

256

CRACKERS

Animal	8–16
Bread sticks	1½ ounces
Cinnamon Crisp (smallest score)	4–6
Cocoa grahams	3–6
Holland rusk	1–2
Honey grahams (smallest score)	4–6
Matzoh (6-inch square)	1–1½
Melba toast	6
Oyster	25–30
Peanut butter or cheese-sandwich type (⅞ ounce)	1 pkg.
Pretzels:	Dutch or soft
	1
3 ring	6–12
Veri-thin—¾ ounce	70–80
Round thin	7
Rye Krisp	3
Saltines	5–8
Sea toast	1–2
Soda	3–6
Triscuit	4–6
Zwieback	3–6

ICE CREAM AND DESSERTS

Chocolate-covered ice cream bar	1
Chocolate-covered ice milk bar	1
Fudge bar	1–2
Ice cream, Chocolate, vanilla, strawberry	¾ cup
Ice milk	¾ cup
Ice cream cone	1
Twin Popsicle	1
Ice cream sandwich (reg. size)	1
Orange cream bar	1
Sherbet	⅔ cup
Toffee crunch bar	1
Water ice	½ cup
Jello	¾ cup

DESSERTS AND SNACKS

Have at least the amount specified. There are no restrictions. If you feel like more, help yourself. Consult your cookbooks for suggestions.

Cheese Tid Bits	50
Fritos	1–2 ounces
Pizza pie, frozen (6-inch)	1
Pizza pie (Chef Boy-ar-dee)	¼
Popcorn	1½ cup

⅙ of an 8-inch pie, any kind, as—

Apple	Lemon meringue
Blueberry	Coconut custard
Cherry	Custard
Mince	Chocolate
Peach	Butterscotch
Pear and grape	Pumpkin
Strawberry	Sweet potato
Blackberry	Apple, cherry, pineapple crumb

1/12 of an 8-inch cake with frosting, as—

Devil's food	Marble
Coconut	Pound
Caramel	Bundt

3 cookies (at least 2 inches in diameter) as—

Oatmeal	Brownies, 2 X 3 inches
Ice box	Date bars, 2 X 3 inches
Sugar	Chocolate drop
Peanut Butter	Macaroons
Chocolate chip	

Puddings—½ cup of chocolate, vanilla, butterscotch, tapioca, baked or boiled custard, plum pudding, cheesecake.

Ice Cream or sherbet, ½ cup any flavor, sundaes

Drinks:

1 cup of malted milk
   milk shake
   soda with ice cream
1 envelope Instant Breakfast made with 1 cup whole milk

Good eating!

A WEEK OF MENU PLANS FOR EASY, NO-RISK WEIGHT-GAIN DIET

[Note: Eat at least this much food; eat more if you like; more if you can. Space your meals at least 3½ to 4 hours apart.]

DAY ONE

Breakfast
½ cup orange juice or more if you wish
¾ cup cornflakes
1 egg, poached
1 slice toast
1 teaspoon butter or margarine
1 teaspoon your favorite jelly
1 cup whole milk
Coffee or tea if desired; sugar and cream as desired

Lunch
(Jumbo) hamburger patty on bun
Tossed salad with mayonnaise or coleslaw
Fresh apple
1 cup milk (whole)
Coffee or tea if desired; sugar and cream as desired

Dinner
2 double lamb chops, broiled
1 large baked potato—sour cream or butter, or margarine
Sliced tomato and cucumber on lettuce with mayonnaise
1 slice chocolate cake with icing
Coffee or tea if desired; sugar and cream as desired

Snack
1 cup milk
1 slice bread with 1 teaspoon butter
                      1 tablespoon peanut butter
                      1 teaspoon jelly or honey

Breakfast ½ cup grapefruit juice
2 waffles (5 inches in diameter) with butter or
margarine and syrup
2 slices crisp bacon
1 cup milk
Coffee or tea if desired; sugar and cream as desired

Lunch Grilled ham and cheese sandwich
Potato chips
Celery sticks and olives
Canned pineapple slices
1 cup milk
Coffee or tea if desired; sugar and cream as desired

Dinner Chianti, if desired
Lasagna—at least 4-ounce serving
Tossed salad with vinegar and oil dressing
Garlic bread
Spumoni
Coffee or tea if desired; sugar and cream as desired

Snack 1 cup milk
2 graham crackers

DAY THREE

Breakfast ¾ cup orange juice
2 eggs scrambled (with cream)
2 link sausages
2 slices toast
2 teaspoons butter or margarine
2 teaspoons orange marmalade
1 cup milk
Coffee or tea if desired; sugar and cream as desired

Lunch Avocado stuffed with shrimp salad on lettuce
French bread with sweet butter (2 slices)
Vanilla ice cream with strawberry sauce
Coffee or tea if desired; sugar and cream as desired

Dinner Cocktail
Roast beef—4 ounces minimum—au jus
Scalloped potatoes
Buttered peas and mushrooms
Relishes
Hot rolls and butter
Baked apple with whipped topping or hard sauce
Coffee or tea if desired; sugar and cream as desired

Snack 1 cup whole milk with 1 envelope of Carnation Slender or similar product

Or, if you prefer, make yourself a nice milk shake with milk, ice cream, and your favorite flavoring.

DAY FOUR

Breakfast   ¾ cup pineapple juice
¾ cup puffed wheat
1 cup milk
1 fried egg
Sweet roll (with butter)
Coffee or tea if desired; sugar and cream as desired

Lunch   Cream of pea soup with croutons
Tuna salad sandwich
1 cup milk
1 piece lemon meringue pie

Mid-afternoon   Ice cream cone or sandwich

Dinner   Chicken stew with dumplings
Asparagus spears with butter
Mixed fruit salad with mayonnaise and coconut
Brownie
1 cup milk
Coffee or tea if desired; sugar and cream as desired

Snack   1 cup milk
Brownie

DAY FIVE

Breakfast ½ grapefruit with honey or sugar
3 pancakes 4 inches in diameter with butter and maple syrup
2 sausage links
1 cup milk
Coffee or tea if desired; sugar and cream as desired

Lunch Chicken salad sandwich
Potato chips
Mixed fruit salad with honey dressing
Chocolate cake
1 cup milk
Coffee or tea if desired; sugar and cream as desired

Dinner Stuffed pork chops
Mashed potatoes
Buttered spinach with hard-cooked egg slices
Lettuce heart with Thousand Island dressing
Hot rolls, butter
Cherry cheesecake
Coffee or tea if desired; sugar and cream as desired

Snack Milk shake—your favorite flavor
(Try 1 cup milk, plus ½ cup your favorite ice cream in the blender. Whiz until your consistency is reached. A couple of graham crackers will be good too.)

DAY SIX

Breakfast ¾ cup orange juice
1 cup oatmeal with brown sugar
1 cup milk
2 eggs scrambled
2 strips of bacon
1 slice toast with butter
1 teaspoon your favorite jelly
Coffee or tea if desired; sugar and cream as desired

Lunch Cream of mushroom soup
Submarine sandwich
Coleslaw
1 cup milk
Canned pineapple slices

Mid-afternoon Chocolate ice cream soda—or your favorite flavor

Dinner Cocktail if you wish
Sugar glazed baked ham
Candied sweet potatoes
Brussels sprouts with lemon butter
Waldorf salad on lettuce
Hot roll and butter or oleo
1 cup milk
Vanilla custard
Coffee or tea if desired; sugar and cream as desired

Snack 1 cup milk
½ ham sandwich

DAY SEVEN

Breakfast 1 fresh orange, sliced
¾ cup Rice Krispies with sugar
1 cup milk
1 poached egg on toast
Butter or margarine
2 slices crisp bacon
Coffee or tea if desired; sugar and cream as desired

Lunch Creamed chipped beef on toast
Mixed citrus fruit salad with coconut and honey dressing
1 cup milk
Peach pie

Mid-afternoon 1 cup milk and 4 cookies—your favorites

Dinner Cocktail if desired
Maryland fried chicken with cream gravy
Mashed potatoes
Buttered carrots and onions
Tossed green salad with blue cheese dressing
Hot rolls and butter or oleo
Pineapple upside-down cake
Coffee or tea if desired; sugar and cream as desired

Snack 1 cup milk
Cereal with sugar or 1 piece peach pie

Now you are ready to increase your intake of food and to continue the increase in weight. Remember, three meals a day are a must; one snack is also a must, either in afternoon or evening or both.

Of the fifty-seven thin people who tried this diet, forty-eight gained an average of four pounds a month. They gained because of one reason—they ate more food.

The nine people who just didn't want to go on a weight-gain diet also successfully gained weight, simply by slightly increasing the size serving of the foods they liked best. They never skipped meals (thin, nervous people often do so when faced with a crisis). They also included snacks, just like meals, but their snacks were neither so large nor so close to their next meal as to destroy their appetite. An afternoon tea time snack *and* a bedtime snack worked well for many people—just so long as the foods they snacked were not junk foods such as pastry, but good wholesome foods of which muscle is made.

If you really don't want to change your eating habits and only want to gain about ten pounds a year, then I have an easy solution for you. Eat as you are eating now. Don't change your daily activities. Just add a large apple, or drink an eight-ounce glass of orange juice each and every day. At the end of the year, you will have gained your ten pounds!

AFTERWORD

The best feeling you can have is the satisfaction that you've succeeded in something important you set out to do. It is that special feeling of knowing you worked diligently, gave it your all, and are proud of your accomplishment.

It is that way with dieting and being healthy. It makes you feel really good to know that you're doing all you can to give your body good nutrition in the right amount for your proper weight.

Eating to lose weight, eating to gain weight, or eating right to keep your figure at its ideal weight, you will find that the discipline you use to arrive at your goal, once set in motion, will keep on working for you—overtime—making you more beautiful on the outside as well as stronger and more confident on the inside. Success will lead to success. Hang in there!

BIBLIOGRAPHY

(For further reading, see *s)

ABC's of Good Nutrition. Department of Health and Mental Hygiene, 1971.

Agricultural Handbook Number 8—Composition of Foods—Raw, Processed, Prepared. Agricultural Research Services, U.S.D.A., Washington, D.C. 1963.

Air Force Diet. Toronto, Air Force Diet Publishers, 1960.

ALLEN, E. WILLIAM, BRENNAN, MILDRED T., HERRON, ARTHUR L., JR., and SELTZER, HOLBROOKE S., "Insulin Secretion in Response to Glycemic Stimulus: Relation of Delayed Initial Release to Carbohydrate Intolerance in Mild Diabetes Mellitus." *Journal of Clinical Investigation,* Vol. 46, No. 3, 1967, pp. 323-335.

AMA Drug Evaluations, 1st ed. Chicago, American Medical Association, 1971.

"AMA Panel Denounces 'Dr. Atkins' Diet Revolution.'" *American Medical News,* March 19, 1973.

The American Heart Association Cookbook. New York, David McKay, 1973.*

ASHER, W. L., "Bariatrics: Struggling for Recognition." *Medical Opinion,* I: 20, 1972.

ATKINS, R. C., *Dr. Atkins' Diet Revolution: The High Calorie Way to Stay Thin Forever*. New York, David McKay, 1972.

AZAR, G. J., and BLOOM, W. L., "Similarities of Carbohydrate Deficiency and Fasting. II. Ketones, Nonesterified Fatty Acids, and Nitrogen Excretion." *Archives of Internal Medicine*, 112: pp. 338-343, 1963.

BANTING, W., *Letter on Corpulence, Addressed to the Public*, 2nd ed. London, Harrison, 1863.

BERLAND, T., "Rating the Diets." *Consumer Guide*, 53, 1974.

BERMAN, EDITH, Personal Communication, January, 1974.

Better Homes and Gardens' Eat and Stay Slim. New York, Meredith Press, 1968.

BLAKESLEE, A., and STAMLER, J., *Your Heart Has Nine Lives: Nine Steps to Heart Health*. Prentice-Hall, 1963.

BLOOM, W. L., "Inhibition of Salt Excretion by Carbohydrate." *Archives of Internal Medicine*, 109: pp. 26-32, 1962.

———, and AZAR, G. J., "Similarities of Carbohydrate Deficiency and Fasting. I. Weight Loss, Electrolyte Excretion, and Fatigue." *Archives of Internal Medicine, 112: 333-337*.

"*Body Images—the Happy American Body: A Survey Report.*" *Psychology Today* (November, 1973), pp. 119-131.

BOWES, ANNA, DE PLANTER, and CHURCH, CHARLES, *Food Values of Portions Commonly Used*, Revised 11th ed. Philadelphia, J.P. Lippincott Co., 1972.

BROWN, D. F., KINCH, S. H., and DOYLE, J. T., "Serum Triglycerides in Health and in Ischemic Heart Disease." *New England Journal of Medicine*, 273: pp. 947-952, 1965.

BRUCH, HILDE, *Eating Disorders*. New York, Basic Books, 1973.

BRUNZELL, J. D., PORTE, D., JR., and BIERMAN, E. L., "Evidence for a Common Saturable Removal System for Removal of Dietary and Endogenous Triglyceride in Man." *Journal of Clinical Investigation*, 50: 15a Abstract 48, 1971.

BUCHWALD, HENRY, MD, PhD, "Jejuno-Ilea Surgery: Which Patients Qualify?" *Medical Opinion*, 2: 40-48 (August, 1973).

———, SCHWARTZ, MARSHALL, MD, and VARCO, RICHARD L., MD, PhD, "Preoperative Preparation, Operative Technique and Postoperative Care of Patients Undergoing Jejunoileal Bypass for Massive Exogenous Obesity." *Journal of Surgical Research*, 147-150 (1973).

Bulletin of the Walter Kempner Foundation, Vol. 4, No. 1. Durham, North Carolina (June, 1972).

CAHILL, G. F., JR., "Physiology of Insulin in Man." *Diabetes*, 20: 785, 1971.

CHANEY, M. S. and ROSS, M. L., *Nutrition*. Boston, Houghton Mifflin, 1971.

CHRISTAKIS, G., *et al.*, "Effect of a Cholesterol-Lowering Diet on Fatty Acid Composition of Subcutaneous Fat in Man." *Circulation*, 26: 648, 1962.

CONNOR, W. E., "Effect of Dietary Lipids upon Chylomicron Composition in Man." *Federation Proceedings*, 18: 473, Abstract 1861, 1959.

———, and HODGES, R. E., and BLEILER, R. E., "The Serum Lipids in Men Receiving High Cholesterol and Cholesterol-Free Diets." *Journal of Clinical Investigation*, 40: 894-901, 1961.

"Course in Gastroenterology." *Mayo Clinic Proceedings*, 48: 620-629 (September, 1973).

"A Critique of Low-Carbohydrate Ketogenic Weight Reduction Regimens—A Review of Dr. Atkins' Diet Revolution." Council of Food and Nutrition of the American Medical Association, JAMA (June 4, 1973).*

CRENSHAW, MARY ANNE, "My Amazing Cider Vinegar, Lecithin, Kelp, B6 Diet, *Family Circle* (January, 1974).

DEAN, RICHARD, MD, SCOTT, H. WILLIAM, JR., MD, *et al.*, "New Considerations in Use of Jejunoileal Bypass in Patients with Morbid Obesity." *Annals of Surgery*, Vol. 177, No. 6 (June, 1973).

DEUEL, H. J., JR., and GULICK, M., "Studies on Ketosis, 1. The Sexual Variation in Starvation Ketosis." *Journal of Biological Chemistry*, 96: 25-34, 1932.

DEUTSCH, R., *Grass Lovers*. New York, Doubleday, 1962.

DEUTSCH, RONALD M., *The Family Guide to Better Food & Better Health*. Des Moines, Better Homes & Garden Books, 1971.

DE VILLE, M., *The Digital Dieters Handbook (originally published as The Remarkable Ratio Diet)*. Denville, New Jersey, Hartford Publishing Corporation, 1973.

"Diet and Heart Disease." American Medical Association news release dated October 8, 1973.*

"Diet Revolution Author is Sued for $7 Million on Heart Attack." New York *Times* (March 23, 1973). Reprinted in *Nutrition and Diseases*, 1973, *op. cit.*, p. 66.

DUPERTUIS, C. WESLEY (Professor Clinical Anthropology, Care Western Reserve University School of Medicine), Personal Communication, April, 1974.

EVANS, J. T., *et al.*, "Superior Vena Cava Obstruction with Substernal Thyroid." *Southern Medical Journal,* 67, No. 1: 3 (January, 1974).

FARBISZERSKI, R., and WOROWSKI, K., "Enhancement of Platelet. Aggregation and Adhesiveness by Beta Lipoprotein." *Journal of Atherosclerosis Research,* 8: 988-990, 1968.

FOLIN, O., and DENIS, W., "On Starvation and Obesity, with Special Reference to Acidosis." *Journal of Biological Chemistry,* 21: 183-192, 1915.

FOMON, S. J., *Infant Nutrition.* Philadelphia, W. B. Saunders, 1967.

Food and Nutrition Board, National Academy of Sciences, National Research Council.

FRANCES, EVAN, *Ladies Home Journal Family Diet Book.* New York, Macmillan Publishing Company, Inc., 1973.

FRIEDMAN, MEYER, and ROSEMAN, RAY H., *Type A Behavior and Your Heart.* New York, Alfred A. Knopf, 1974.

GAMBLE, J. L., ROSS, G. S., and TISDALL, R. R., "The Metabolism of Fixed Base During Fasting." *Journal of Biological Chemistry,* 57: 633-695, 1923.

GHARIB, HOSSEIN, "Triiodothyronine, Physiological and Clinical Significance." Journal of the American Medical Association, 227, No. 3: 302 (January 21, 1974).

GRANDE, R., "Energy Balance and Body Composition Changes: A Critical Study of Three Recent Publications." *Annals of Internal Medicine,* 68: 467-480, 1968.

GREIG, H. B. W., "Inhibition of Fibrinolysis by Alimentary Lipaemia." *Lancet,* 2, 16-18, 1956.

GUILFORD, CAROL, *The Diet Book.* New York, Pinnacle Books, 1973.

HARRIS, HELEN, "How to Cope with Wrinkles & Crinkles, Flab and Sag You Don't Want," *Harper's Bazaar* (April, 1974), p. 43.

HARVEY, W., *On Corpulence in Relation to Disease.* London, Henry Renshaw, 1872.

HAUSER, GAYELORD, *The New Diet Does It.* New York, Berkley Books, 1972.

The Healthy Way to Weigh Less. Chicago, American Medical Association, 1973.

HERVEY, G. R., and MCCANCE, R. A., "The Effects of Carbohydrate and Sea Water on the Metabolism of Men Without

Food or Sufficient Water." *Proceedings of the Royal Society* (Biol) 139: 527-545, 1952.

HOAK, J. C., CONNOR, W. E., and WARNER, E. D., "Toxic Effects of Glucagon-Induced Acute Lipid Mobilization in Geese." *Journal of Clinical Investigation*, 47: 2701-2710, 1968.

————, "Effects of Acute Free Fatty Acid Mobilization on the Heart," in BAJUSZ, E., and RONA, G., Eds., *Myocardiology: Recent Advances in Studies of Cardiac Structure and Metabolism*, Vol. 1. Baltimore, University Park Press, 1972.

HOWARD, PAMELA, and TREADWELL, SANDY, "Dr. Atkins Says He's Sorry." *New York*, March 26, 1973. Reprinted in *Nutrition and Diseases*—1973, Hearing Before the Select Committee on Nutrition and Human Needs of the U.S. Senate, 93rd Congress, April 12, 1973. Washington: USGPO, Stock No. 5270-01835. 1973.*

HUBBARD, T. BRANNON, JR., MD, Mercy Hospital, Baltimore, Personal communication, December, 1973.

INGELFINGER, FRANZ J., MD, "Regional Absorption." *American Journal of Surgery* (September, 1967), pp. 388-392.

"In Obesity Surgery, Problems are the Rule." *Medical World News* (September 7, 1973), pp. 34, 35.

INSULL, W., OISO, I., and TSUCHIYA, K., "Diet and Nutritional Status of Japanese." *American Journal of Clinical Nutrition*, 21: 753-777, 1968.

JAMESON, G., and WILLIAMS, E., *The Drinking Man's Diet*. San Francisco, Cameron and Co., 1964.

KANNEL, W. B., *et al.*, "Serum Cholesterol, Lipoproteins, and the Risk of Coronary Heart Disease: The Framingham Study." *Annals of Internal Medicine*, 74: 1-12, 1971.

KAPILOFF, BERNARD, MD Personal Communication, January, 1974.

KEKWICK, A., and PAWAN, G. L. S., "Calorie Intake in Relation to Body Weight Changes in the Obese." *Lancet*, 2: 155-161, 1956.

KELLY, THOMAS R., MD, KLEIN, ROBERT L., MD, and WOODFORD, JAMES W., MD, "Alterations in Gallstone Solubility Following Distal Ileal Resection." *Archives of Surgery*, Vol. 105 (August, 1972), pp. 352-355.

KEYS, ANCEL, and MARGARET, *Eat Well and Stay Well*. Garden City, New York, Doubleday, 1963.*

KONISH, FRANK, *Exercise Equivalents of Foods*. Carbondale, Southern Illinois University Press, 1974.

273

KRAUS, BARBARA, *A Dictionary of Calories and Carbohydrates.* New York, Grosset & Dunlap, 1973.

LAMB, LAWRENCE E., *What You Need to Know About Food and Cooking for Health.* New York, Viking, 1973.

LASAGNA, LOUIS, "Attitudes Toward Appetite Suppressants." *Journal of the American Medical Association,* 225: 44-48 (July 2, 1973). *

LAW, DAVID H., MD, SCOTT, H. WILLIAM, JR., MD, *et al.*, "Jejunoileal Shunt in Surgical Treatment of Morbid Obesity." *Annals of Surgery,* Vol. 171, No. 5 (May, 1970).

LEVERTON, RUTH, *Food Becomes You.* Ames, Iowa State University, 1965.

LEVITSKY, D., "Regulation of Adiposity and the Control of Food Intake." Presented at the first annual meeting of the American Society of Clinical Nutrition and American Institute of Nutrition, at Cornell University, August 14-17, 1973.

LEWIS, LENA A., PhD, PAGE, IRVING H., MD, and TURNBULL, RUPERT B., JR., MD, "'Short-Circuiting' of the Small Intestine— Effect on Concentration of Serum Cholesterol and Lipoproteins." *Journal of the American Medical Association,* Vol. 182, No. 1 (October 6, 1962), pp. 77-79.

LINCOLN, JETSON E., "Calorie Intake, Obesity, and Physical Activity." *American Journal of Clinical Nutrition,* 25: 390-394 (April, 1972).

LINDAUER, LOIS LYONS, Personal communication, March, 1974.

————, *It's In to be Thin.* New York, Award Books, 1970.

LINDER, PETER G., *Mind Over Platter.* North Hollywood, California, Wilshire Book Co., 1972.

LOCKWOOD, DEAN, MD, Johns Hopkins Hospital, Baltimore, Personal communication, December, 1973.

LUSK, G., *The Elements of the Science of Nutrition.* New York, W. B. Saunders Company, 1906.

MACBRYDE, CYRIL M., MD, FACP, "The Diagnosis of Obesity." *Medical Clinics of North America,* Vol. 48, 1964, pp. 1307-1316.

MANN, GEORGE V., "Obesity, the Nutritional Spook." *American Journal of Public Health,* 61: 1491-1498 (August, 1971).*

Manual of Applied Nutrition, The Johns Hopkins Hospital Nutrition Dept. Janette Carlsen, Chairman of Revision Committee. Sixth Edition, 1973. The Johns Hopkins Press, Baltimore, and London, England.*

MART, DONALD S., *The Carbo-Calorie Diet.* Garden City, New York, Doubleday, 1973.

MAYER, JEAN, "Bazaar's Super Salad Diet," *Harper's Bazaar* (April, 1974), p. 44.

MAYER, JEAN, —— *Overweight.* Englewood Cliffs, New Jersey, Prentice-Hall, 1968.

——, "Why Exercise Pays." *Blue Print for Health,* 24: 10-17, 1973, Blue Cross Association, Chicago.*

MCCLELLAN, W. W., and DUBOIS, E. F., "Prolonged Meat Diets with a Study of Kidney Function and Ketosis." *Journal of Biological Chemistry,* 87: 651-668, 1930.

MCLAREN, D. S., and PELLET, P. L., "Nutrition in the Middle East," in BOURNE, G. J., Ed., *World Review of Nutrition and Dietetics,* Vol. 12. Basel, Switzerland, S. Karger, 1970, pp. 43-127.

MCMAHON, ED, *Slimming Down.* New York, Grosset & Dunlap, 1972.

MCWILLIAMS, M., *Nutrition for the Growing Years.* New York, John Wiley, 1967.

Meal Planning with Exchange Lists. Committees of American Diabetes Association, Inc., and The American Dietetic Association in cooperation with Chronic Disease Program—Public Health Service Department of Health, Education and Welfare.*

Mealtime Manual for the Aged and Handicapped. Institute of Rehabilitation, New York University Medical Center. Simon & Schuster, 1970.

The Medical Society of the County of New York, Personal communication, January, 1974.

MERIGAN, T. C., *et al.,* "Effect of Chylomicrons on Fibrinolytic Activity of Normal Human Plasma in Vitro." *Circulation Research,* 7: 205-209, 1959.

MONELLO, LENORE F., MD, and MAYER, JEAN, PhD, DSc, "Obese Adolescent Girls: An Unrecognized 'Minority ' Group?" *American Journal of Clinical Nutrition,* Vol. 13 (July, 1963), pp. 35-39.

NELSON, RALPH A., *et al.,* "Physiology and Natural History of Obesity." *Journal of the American Medical Association,* 223: 627-630, 1973.

"Nutrition and Disease, 1973 Hearings before the Select Committee on Nutrition and Human Needs of the United States Senate, 93rd Congress." Washington, D.C., April 12, 1973.*

"Nutrition and the Elderly, 1973 Hearings before the Select Committee on Nutrition and Human Needs of the United States Senate, 93rd Congress." Washington, D.C., May 30, 1973. *

Nutrition, Why Is It Important? Campbell's Soup Company, December, 1973. *

"Obesity Surgery Aids Four Adolescents." *Medical World News* (November 16, 1973), p. 21.

OLESEN, E. S., and QUAADE, F., "Fatty Foods and Obesity." *Lancet*, 1: 1048-1051, 1960.

OLIVER, M. F., KURIEN, V. A., and GREENWOOD, T. W., "Relation Between Serum-Free Fatty Acids and Arrhythmias and Death after Acute Myocardial Infarction." *Lancet*, 1: 710-714, 1968.

OLIVER, M. T., and YATES, P. A., "Induction of Ventricular Arrhythmias by Elevation of Arterial Free Fatty Acids in Experimental Myocardial Infarction." In MORET, P., and FEIFER, Z., eds., *Metabolism of the Hyposic and Ischaemic Heart*. Basel, Switzerland, S. Karger, 1972, p. 359.

"Once Gained, Seldom Lost." *Medical World News* (October 6, 1972), pp. 63, 66.

PASSMORE, SIR STANLEY D. R., *Human Nutrition and Dietetics*. Baltimore, Williams and Wilkins, 1966.

PAYNE, ALMA S., and CALLAHAN, D., *The Fat and Sodium Control Cookbook*. Boston, Little Brown, 1966.

PAYNE, J. HOWARD, MD, et al., "Metabolic Observations in Patients with Jejunocolic Shunts." *American Journal of Surgery*, Vol. 106 (August, 1963).

PEARSON, LEONARD, PEARSON, LILLIAN R., and SAEKEL, KAROLA, *The Psychologists' Eat-Anything Diet*. New York, David McKay, 1973.

PENNINGTON, A. W., "An Alternate Approach to the Problem of Obesity." *Journal of Clinical Nutrition*, 1: 100-106, 1953.

————, "Treatment of Obesity with Calorically Unrestricted Diets." *Journal of Clinical Nutrition*, 1: 343-348, 1953.

PHILIP, R. B., and WRIGHT, H. P., "Effect of Adenosine on Platelet Adhesiveness in Fasting and Lipaemic Bloods." *Lancet* 2: 208-209. 1965.

PILKINGTON, T. R. E., et al., "Diet and Weight Reduction in the Obese." *Lancet*, 1: 856-858, 1960.

"Primary Prevention of the Atherosclerotic Disease." Inter-Society Commission for Heart Disease Resources, Atherosclerosis and Epidemiology Study Groups. *Circulation*, 42: A-55-A-95, 1970.

PROXMIRE, WILLIAM, *You Can Do It!* New York, Simon and Schuster, 1973.*

"The Prudent Diet: Vintage 1973." *Medical World News* (August 10, 1973), pp. 33-44.*

Recipes for Fat-Controlled, Low Cholesterol Meals. New York, American Heart Association, 1972.

Recommended Dietary Allowances, 8th ed., 1973. National Academy of Sciences, Washington, D.C., 1973.

Reconstructive Plastic Surgery: Principles and Procedures in Correction, Reconstruction, and Transplantation, 5 vols., Jean Marquis Converse, MD, ed. Philadelphia, W.B. Saunders, 1964.

RICHMAN, FRANK; MITCHELL, NANCY; DINGMAN, JOSEPH; and DALEN, JAMES, "Changes in Serum Cholesterol During the Stillman Diet," *JAMA*, Vol. 228, No. 1 (April, 1974).

RONSARD, NICOLA, *Cellulite: Those Lumps, Bumps and Bulges You Couldn't Lose Before.* New York, Beauty and Health Publishing Corp., 1973.

RUBIN, THEODORE ISAAC, *Forever Thin.* New York, Bernard Geis Associates, 1970.

―――, *The Thin Book by a Formerly Fat Psychiatrist.* New York, Pinnacle Books, 1972.

SALMON, PETER A.,MD, FACS, "The Results of Small Intestine Bypass Operations for the Treatment of Obesity." *Surgery, Gynecology and Obstetrics,* Vol. 132, No. 6 (June, 1971).

SCHOENBERG, H., *Cookbook for Calorie Watchers.* New York, Goodhousekeeping Books, 1972.

SCHWARTZ, T. B., and BECKER, F. O., *The Year Book of Endocrinology 1973.* Chicago, Year Book Medical Publishers.

SCOTT, H. WILLIAM, JR., MD, "Intestinal Bypass Operation in Treatment of Massive Obesity." *Hospital Practice,* Vol. 7, No. 11 (November, 1972).

SHIPMAN, WILLIAM G., PhD, "Psychological Aspects of Obesity and Dieting." International Congress of Applied Psychology, Liege, Belgium, July, 1971.

SHOSHKES, M., *et al.,* "Fat Emulsions for Oral Nutrition; Use of Orally Administered Fat Emulsions as Calorie Supplements in Man." *Journal of the American Dietetic Association,* 27: 197-208, 1951.

SIMONSON, MARIA, MD, Behavioral Laboratory, Johns Hopkins

277

School of Hygiene, Personal communication, December, 1973.

Skinfolds, Body Girths, Biacromial Diameter, and Selected Anthropometric Indices of Adults. Washington: USGPO, PHS Pub. No. 1000—Series 11, No. 35, 1970.

SMALL, MARVIN, *The Easy 24 Hour Diet.* Garden City, New York, Doubleday, 1973.

SOLOMON, NEIL, MD, PhD, "Health Hazards of Obesity." *Obesity and Bariatric Medicine,* 1, No. 1: 3-5 (May-June, 1972).

———, "Studying and Treating the Obese Patient." *Maryland State Medical Journal,* 17: 64-69 (May, 1968).

———, "The Study and Treatment of the Obese Patient." *Hospital Practice,* 4: 90-94 (March, 1969).

———, "Weight Loss Through Food Withdrawal." *The Bulletin of the Maryland Dietetic Association,* Vol. 18, No. 2: 3, 1966.

———, CARPENTER, C. G. J., BENNETT, I. L., and HARVEY, A. M., "Schmidt's Syndrome (Thyroid and Adrenal Insufficiency) and the Co-existence of Diabetes Mellitus." *Diabetes,* 14: 300, 1965.

———, and DENDRINOS, GEORGE J., *Current Diagnosis*—Section 9, Disorders of Metabolism—Obesity. Philadelphia-London-Toronto, W. B. Saunders, 1971.

———, and SHEPPARD, SALLY, *The Truth About Weight Control: How to Lose Excess Pounds Permanently.* New York, Stein and Day, 1972.

———, and SHOCK, N. W., "Nutrition in the Aged." *Southern Medical Journal,* 62, No. 12: 1523-28 (December, 1969).

———, "Psychologic Effects of Prolonged Starvation in Extreme Obesity." *Southern Medical Journal,* 63, No. 3: 274-279 (March, 1970).

———, and AUGHENBAUGH, PATRICIA S., "The Daily Needs and Interest of Older People," Chapter 10, *The Biology of Aging.* Fort Lauderdale, Charles C. Thomas, 1970.

———, DAVIDOFF, A., WINKLER, S., and LEE, M. H. M., EDS., *Dentistry for the Special Patient: The Aged, Chronically Ill and Handicapped,* Chapter 2, Physiology of Aging. Philadelphia-London-Toronto, W. B. Saunders, 1972.

STARE, FREDERICK J. (Professor of Nutrition, Chairman, Department of Nutrition, Harvard University), Personal Communication, January, 1974.

———, *Eating for Good Health.* Garden City, New York, Doubleday, 1969.

———, "Overnutrition," *American Journal of Public Health,* 53: 1795-1802 (November, 1963).

————, and WITSCHI, JELIA C., "Diet Books: Facts, Fads and Frauds." *Medical Opinion*, I: 13, 1972.

Statement on Hypoglycemia. Editorial, *Journal of the American Medical Association*, 223: 682, 1973.*

STILLMAN, I. M., and BAKER, S. S., *The Doctor's Quick Weight-Loss Diet*. Englewood Cliffs, New Jersey, Prentice-Hall, 1967.

————, *Doctor Stillman's 14-Day Shape-Up Program*. New York, Delacorte Press, 1974.

————, *The Doctor's Quick Inches-Off Diet*, New York, Dell Books, 1970.

STUNKARD, ALBERT J., "The Success of TOPS, a Self-Help Group." *Postgraduate Medicine* (May, 1972), pp. 143-147.*

————, *et al.*, "Influence of Social Class on Obesity and Thinness in Children." *Journal of the American Medical Association*, 221: 579-584 (August 7, 1972).

"Suit Ties Dr. Atkins' Diet to Heart Attack." *American Medical News* (April 2, 1973), p. 13.

TALLER, H., *Calories Don't Count*. New York, Simon and Schuster, 1961.

TATKON, D., *The Great Vitamin Hoax*. New York, Macmillan, 1968.

TOLSTOI, E., "The Effect of an Exclusive Meat Diet on the Chemical Constituents of the Blood." *Journal of Biological Chemistry*, 83: 753-758, 1929.

"Viewpoint: A Young Scientist's View of Gerontology." *Geriatrics*, 22 (January, 1967).

WALDEN, EMERSON, Personal communication, December, 1973.

"Weighing Pregnancy's Calorie Cost," *Medical World News* (January 12, 1973), p. 86A.

WEISMANN, RODGER E., "Surgical Palliation of Massive and Severe Obesity." *The American Journal of Surgery*, Vol. 125 (April, 1973), pp. 437-446.

WERNER, S. C., "Comparison Between Weight Reduction on a High-Calorie, High Fat Diet and on an Isocaloric Regimen High in Carbohydrate." *New England Journal of Medicine*, 252: 661-665, 1955.

WEST, E. S., *et al.*, *Textbook of Biochemistry*, 4th ed. New York, Macmillan, 1967.

WEST, K. M., and KALBFLEISCH, J. M., "Glucose Tolerance Nutrition, and Diabetes in Uruguay, Venezuela, Malaya and East Pakistan." *Diabetes*, 15: 9-18, 1966.

"When to Start Dieting? At Birth." *Medical World News* (September 7, 1973), pp. 31-33.

WHITE, A., *et al.*, *Principles of Biochemistry*. New York, McGraw-Hill, 1954.

WHITE, PHILIP L., MD (Director, Department of Foods and Nutrition, American Medical Association, Chicago), Personal communication, January, 1974.

————, *Let's Talk About Food*. Chicago, The American Medical Association, 1967.*

WOHL, MICHAEL G., and GOODHARDT, ROBERT S., *Modern Nutrition in Health and Disease*, 4th ed. Philadelphia, Lea and Febiger, 1972.

WYDEN, PETER, *The Overweight Society*. New York, William Morrow, 1965.

————, and WYDEN, BARBARA, *How the Doctors Diet*. New York, Trident, 1968.

————, and LIBIEN, L., *The All-in-One Diet Annual*. New York, Bantam Books, 1970.

YOUNG, J., *The Medical Messiahs*. Princeton, Princeton University Press, 1967.

YUDKIN, J., and CAREY, M., "The Treatment of Obesity by the 'High Fat' Diet. The Inevitability of Calories." *Lancet*, 2: 939-941, 1960.

INDEX